Bodydoctor®

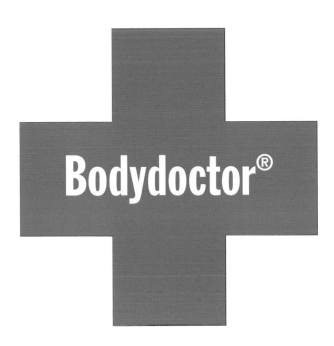

Bodydoctor®

TRUST ME, I'M THE BODYDOCTOR

DAVID MARSHALL

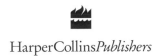

HarperCollins*Publishers*

You should consult your doctor before starting any nutritional
or fitness programme, or if you have any health concerns. The
creators, publishers and distributors of this programme accept
no responsibility for any accident or injury that arises from
performing this programme. Bodydoctor Fitness is a registered
trademark.

HarperCollins*Publishers*
77–85 Fulham Palace Road
Hammersmith, London W6 8JB

The HarperCollins website address is:
www.harpercollins.co.uk

Published by HarperCollins*Publishers* 2004

10 9 8 7 6 5 4

A catalogue record of this book
is available from the British Library

ISBN 0 00 717685 6

Printed and bound in Great Britain by
Butler and Tanner Ltd, Frome and London

CONTENTS

The Bodydoctor team:

Steve Marshall

Steve played rugby for Wasps, represented the county at all age levels, played for London and South-East England at U-18 and U-21 levels, and was selected as a member of the England U-21 squad. Steve qualified as a sports therapist after knee injuries forced him to retire. He has worked at Bodydoctor Fitness for three years.

Sean Durkan, BSc(Hons) Osteopathy

Sean runs a busy and successful osteopathic clinic at 140 Harley Street. Where suitable, the Bodydoctor Fitness Programme forms an integral part of his patient management and treatment.

Amanda Moore

Amanda is a nutritionist with a successful clinical practice in Richmond and at selected health clubs. Amanda works with Bodydoctor Fitness to help clients achieve their health and weight goals.

Jean-Christophe Novelli

Jean-Christophe has been awarded the Michelin star four times since 1992. He has also received the honour of winning several other prestigious awards including Chef's Chef of the Year. In 1996 he opened his first restaurant, Maison Novelli, in Clerkenwell, going on to launch four other restaurants the following year. He is presently chef patron at Auberge du Lac restaurant, Brocket Hall.

Thanks to the entire Bodydoctor team: Steve Marshall; Sean Durkan; Amanda Moore; Jean-Christophe Novelli; Liz Dean, the editor; Guy Hearn, the photographer; all the models in the book: Noel Levy, Roxanne Marshall, Ashley Harvey, Mark Rawlinson and Paul Ellis; and the HarperCollins team: Wanda Whiteley, Simon Gerratt, Natasha Tait, Jacqui Caulton, Emma Williams and Nicole Linhardt.

Many thanks to Amanda Moore for her invaluable contribution to the nutrition section and Jean-Christophe Novelli, Susan Clark and *Tesco Food* magazine for supplying the recipes in Part Three.

PART ONE

IN THE NEXT SIX WEEKS YOU WILL:

- **TAKE UP TO SIX INCHES OFF YOUR WAIST**

- **DOUBLE YOUR FITNESS**

- **LOSE UP TO ONE STONE.**

Are you nodding your head vigorously like one of those dogs in the back of an old Ford Escort? Then stick with me. I promise that you will meet all these objectives — and more besides — if you just follow my programme. Trust me! I'm the Bodydoctor!

SIX WEEKS FROM NOW, YOU WILL BE:

- **STRONGER**
- **FIRMER**
- **SLIMMER**
- **FITTER**

But let's just get one thing straight before we start. The programme works for everybody. It will work if you are overweight, unfit or a former couch potato. It has worked for Hollywood film stars, Premier League footballers, supermodels, businessmen and mothers recovering from childbirth. It will work for you. It does not matter if you are young or old, short or tall, male or female.

YOU JUST HAVE TO DO IT
DON'T THINK ABOUT IT
DON'T TALK ABOUT IT
DO IT

Why trust me?

I've been fit and fat, slim and slob. I've been there and come back. I know the journey, because I made it. I know the Honey Monster, because I grew up with it. I know the feeling of going somewhere and feeling like the fat kid, the one who didn't belong. I know what it's like to go into a room two or three stone overweight.

I thought I had a mountain to climb, but I turned it into a slope. It can be done — I did it, and so have thousands of others... Now it's your turn to get your health, your body and your life back.

If you don't speak from experience, you can't relate. If you've never had anything more fattening or alcoholic than a glass of celery juice, stuffed yourself on more than a few leaves of lettuce, fantasized about a fry-up or had more then 10 per cent body fat and have been so lean that even a hungry wolf wouldn't look at you, how would you know what it's like to be Billy Bunter or Betty Big Bum? You don't. You can't relate to it, you can't understand it, and you certainly can't begin to rectify it. All you know and preach is a theory that went out with the bow and arrow, and I'm telling you that nobody got fit from a blackboard.

When I wouldn't listen to my doctor's advice and played football after an injury, I ended up with a pressure bandage for a whole year. And I did what many of you might be able to relate to: I comfort ate. That's when I really made friends with the Honey Monster. It was a race against time to see how many Jaffa cakes or burgers I could get down. That's what I did, because my dream was over. I just sat there and stuffed my face. I couldn't exactly run around the block, because I had a pressure bandage that stretched from my groin right down to my toes. With an itchy leg and no way to scratch it, I just filled my belly. So that is why I'm qualified to say I know what it's like to be fat and unfit.

You can read how I beat the bulge on page 19. But for now, just know that you can do it too.

For the last four years, tens of thousands of people all over the world have successfully used the Bodydoctor Fitness Programme by mail order.

What this programme can do for you

Asthma sufferers discover that the Bodydoctor Fitness Programme relieves their symptoms. People debilitated by chronic fatigue syndrome (ME) regain the strength to carry on with their day-to-day lives. Diabetics notice that their insulin levels are much easier to control. People with arthritis find that their symptoms are alleviated. Those crippled with back pain improve their mobility as their related muscles get lean and strong. I even had a client recovering from triple heart-bypass surgery who claimed that the programme sped up his rehabilitation. I could go on.

I am not claiming that I have discovered a miracle cure, but over the past 10 years Bodydoctor clients have experienced some unexpected but welcome side effects. (Read their stories and judge for yourself – see pages 8–11 and 22–65). Yet what makes this even more surprising is that everybody follows the same programme. One size definitely fits all.

That is not as strange as it sounds. After all, everybody has the same physiology. That's how I know this programme will work for you. And your friends.

The Bodydoctor Fitness Programme works because I know that it's the only exercise and nutritional system designed to put your body back into balance. So how does it work?

Get your body back into balance

I have noticed that other exercise programmes promise to make you lose weight, or improve strength or endurance. They rarely promise to achieve all these simultaneously. But I believe that targeting one particular area merely creates imbalances in your body. And these imbalances can lead to major problems.

Imagine the body as a tree. For it to be healthy, you need a strong trunk before you can start putting pressure on the branches. All the exercises in my programme have been chosen to make your trunk strong, yet flexible. These are called 'core' exercises. When you have a strong, healthy and fit core within your body, you can achieve anything.

A sharp mind and a healthy body go hand in hand. Whether you're a celebrity on the climb to stardom or you're just trying to get your two kids and shopping up to the eighteenth floor, you need adequate resources to deal with the pressure. A healthy body gives you better protection against every kind of stress, both mental and physical.

Even professional athletes have their strengths and weaknesses. Most people tend to concentrate on their strengths, and accept their weaknesses. That's human nature! Unfortunately, it means that their strengths are magnified, but the weaknesses are not addressed. Occasionally weaknesses may improve, but generally this is an unexpected side effect. Ultimately, the gap between our strengths and weaknesses becomes vast, bringing increased vulnerability to injury and illness.

Working with your body

When the body embarks on an exercise regime, it can respond in one of two ways. It can enjoy it, or it can recoil in shock and get stiff and sore. It will ache. This is your body's way of indicating that it doesn't like what you are doing to it. The regime just doesn't feel natural, so it does what it can to restrict the movements. It is just the body's way to protect itself.

The Bodydoctor Fitness Programme works with your body – not with some of it, but all of it. And, strange though it may seem, this actually turns conventional exercise wisdom on its head. I don't advocate working on your chest one day, arms the next and belly some time later in the week as other trainers might. This programme works the whole body. Every time you follow it, every single muscle group is activated.

Any exercise creates a positive and negative reaction. Take the chest pressing exercise, for example, which is the third exercise in my programme (see page 92 or 122). As you push the weights, the pectoral muscles in your body contract. The body, naturally, then wants to expand them. In other words, your body's inclination is to stretch. But most exercise regimes ignore this and instead include a whole series of sequential contraction exercises without ever paying attention to what the body desires during the workout itself. Usually, the stretching only comes right at the end of a session, when I believe it is too late; the damage has already been done. In the Bodydoctor Fitness Programme, you stretch and clean your muscles as you work through the exercises (see page 77) – for example, the chest press is immediately followed by an adapted pull-over. This has a secondary effect of stretching out the pectoral muscles, which are still contracted from the chest press. The exercise acts as a counterbalance to its predecessor, but it also has another primary purpose. The pull-over works your back, shoulders and arms. It has a dual function. You also stretch after you've finished the abdominal workout (see page 148) and there's a set of flexibility exercises at the end of the sequence (see page 178).

Now some chefs may not mind if you play around with their recipes and throw in some extra ingredients, but I do. The Bodydoctor Fitness Programme is a series of sequential exercises. They are not laid out in the book to look pretty. They are set out for a reason. You must follow the exact sequence. An exercise that contracts a muscle is immediately followed by one that stretches it. I call this 'cleaning as you go'.

How many times have you been to an exercise class, worked hard and then the next day struggled to get out of bed? That should not happen with the Bodydoctor Fitness Programme. Okay, there may initially be some mild discomfort – after all, you might be working muscles that have probably been inactive for years – but it will not be debilitating. And I promise you that within a short period these minor aches will disappear. You will progress to working with heavier weights, and your body will not even flinch. Soon you'll look back with astonishment at the small weights you first trained with.

True fitness is having a body that is strong, flexible and powerful. It should be able to perform a full spectrum of requirements. It is no good being able to run a mile after a bus if, when you get on board, you can't keep your balance; or looking like an Olympic gold medallist if you are unable to climb two flights of stairs without getting out of breath.

Do this workout 3 times a week or every other day if you prefer. (Up to 5 times a week is perfectly safe as you are using light weights.)

This book will save and change your life — but no one ever got fit and healthy sitting on their bum reading about it. This book gives you the tools and the knowledge. All you need do now is make the decision to follow the programme. No one else will do it for you. You've spent your money — so what have you got to lose but lard?

A tale of three ladies

The following case studies were commissioned for an article by a leading national newspaper. For some reason, it was never published (if the editor is reading this, perhaps they could let me know why. My private view is that the programme demonstrated such success that it seemed too good to be true!)

I was asked to train three women to prove that the Bodydoctor Fitness Programme works for all age groups: one in her early thirties, one approaching 40 and one in her fifties (although you wouldn't think it!). They all started training in the middle of October, which took them up to the middle of December. It was the party season, yet they all achieved successful inch loss. Don't just take my word for it. Read their stories!

And do you know what? They followed exactly the same programme that you're about to start!

Lisa Gorman

Lisa Gorman is 33. She's a photographer's agent, running her own agency in Covent Garden. She lives in King's Cross, London, and is single. After completing the programme, Lisa went down two dress sizes.

'My best friend is the actress and model, Patricia Velasquez, who was staying with me when she was shooting The Mummy Returns in London. She had to be really fit for the fight scenes in her film. Within three weeks, she transformed before my eyes. It was unbelievable. She had a great body anyway (after all, she is a model) and has done the Chanel campaign, but within a month her body had completely changed shape. It was much more defined. I was so impressed that I went to see David and, after speaking to him, I decided I would do the course.

I'm 10 stone and have never been fat, but I wanted to be toned. I've always been fit, but I felt that I'd let my fitness levels go a bit.

After just six sessions with David, my body started changing dramatically. I've done weight training before and worked with personal fitness trainers in the past; I even used to run marathons for charity. But I've never done anything like this. You get individual attention. There are never more than three people in the gym at one time.

There's a massive difference between David's routine and other routines. For a start, you do the same routine every time. Other trainers tend to concentrate on your upper body one day and your lower body the next. But here, you work all the muscles every time you go. I was surprised at how basic the routines are, but they create such change – even using the same machines that you see in a regular gym. There's no high-tech equipment, just different methods of using the regular machines.

I was struck by the precision of each exercise. You are told exactly how to position yourself, how to hold a weight. The difference between the right way and the wrong way can be a matter of just a few degrees. And the Bodydoctor trainers watch you like a hawk. They just don't allow you to go wrong. In other gyms, there isn't the same motivation to succeed. Here, you concentrate so much more. David doesn't even allow music, because he says you should be focussing on the work.

The sessions are very hard work and the trainers really push you. But they made me get through it. David's a real character; he's determined, so he makes you more determined. He believes 100 per cent in what he's doing. It's tough doing one-and-a-half hours' intensive exercise, three times a week. Despite the fact that it was such hard work, I felt very fit from the start of the six weeks and not at all tired.

By the end of the programme I'd gone down two sizes. I was a generous size 12 before, but now a 10 is big on me. The fat's just fallen off me, and it seems like I've shrunk. I'm much more defined all over, especially on my legs and waist. My abdomen is really toned and I'm delighted to see that I even have dips at either side. In the summer, my trousers were tight. Now they're hanging off me.

Emily Foden

Emily Foden is 39 years old and lives in Clapham Common, South London. She is married with two children and runs a catering business with her husband. After the course, she lost 35 per cent of her body fat.

'I used to be very slim, but then I had two children – and it all went horribly wrong. Before the children, I had always been a size 10. Then, as I approached 40, I went up to a size 14–16. I think that having my own business slowed everything down. I just wasn't making the time to go to the gym, which was a shame because I used to be very fit. When I went to David, my dream was to get into a size-10 dress and improve my fitness levels.

I tried two personal trainers before I started the course with David. One of them was based in a gym and I used to work out with weights, but I didn't notice much difference in my shape and lost motivation to keep it up. The other trainer was much more outdoorsy. We used to run around the park. But I got shin splints from running on the grass so much.

I read about Bodydoctor Fitness two years ago and kept the article. Then this year I eventually followed it up. When I started with David I was surprised to find that the routine was the same every time. There is no variation, whereas other trainers had taught me to focus on different areas on different days. This is much more consistent and precise.

I found some of the equipment difficult at first, especially the Stairmaster Crossrobic, which I still find hard. I followed David's eating plan, which is based on the food-combining principle, as well as I could. Given that I work in the catering business, it was quite difficult but I usually managed to have a protein meal midday and a carbohydrate meal in the evening.

In the first week, my energy levels were soaring and I felt fitter than I had done in ages. In two to three weeks, I noticed a considerable difference in my overall fitness. After four weeks my clothes started to feel loose and people were telling me that I'd lost weight, especially on my face.

I actually missed some of my sessions due to work commitments, and so didn't get the full benefits of the course. David tells me that I would have noticed even more of a difference had I not missed those sessions. But despite that, I'm delighted with the results. Now my clothes are very loose. I've gone down to a size 10–12. My stomach has got flatter and everybody tells me that I look much thinner, but well with it. My husband says that my whole shape has changed. But then he knows he'd get his ears boxed if he didn't.

Michelle Carter

Michelle Carter is 56 years old and 4 ft 11 in (1.5 m). She weighed 8 stone 10 lbs (55.3 kilos) when she started the course. By the end of the course, she had lost one third of her body fat. She lost 16½ in (41cm) overall, including 6½ in (16 cm) from her waist.

At 4 ft 11 in, I'm quite a tiny person. Even though I'm 56, I'm as sensitive and concerned about my appearance as I was when I was a teenager. I'd feel ashamed when walking into a cocktail party because, at my height, it doesn't matter how dressed up you are. You look unattractive if you're carrying excess weight. I was a size 12 bordering on a 14, which looked huge on my frame. Ideally, I like to be small, neat and compact.

Like most women, I've been on one diet or another since I was 16. Until I came to see the Bodydoctor, I'd lost hope. I've tried half-a-dozen dieticians and 10 personal trainers, but never achieved weight loss and just ended up hurting myself. I spent four years and a lot of money with one trainer, religiously following her regime, but there was no change in the way I looked. One trainer I tried was actually recommended to me because he specializes in training injured or weak people, but I ended up hurting my back. Another made me over-exercise beyond my body's capabilities at a time when I was not strong at all. I ended up with pulled muscles. I honestly believed nothing, short of surgery, would help me lose weight.

I read about the Bodydoctor some time ago, but past experience had made me sceptical and I didn't want to commit to spending any more money on fitness. Last year I was feeling very low. I couldn't buy the clothes I liked as they didn't fit me. My husband described me as being on the wrong side of chubby.

I decided to take the risk and started an intensive course with the Bodydoctor.

For the first couple of weeks, I was absolutely shattered after sessions at the gym and would go home to bed. I had to do my shopping and chores on non-gym days. It was actually David who suspected that something was wrong and sent me to a nutritionist who diagnosed low blood pressure. I changed my diet according to David's eating plan, and persevered with the workouts.

Gradually, I began to feel fitter and stronger. Because it's a very easy routine the body adjusts, and it feels that the muscles are being worked in the right order. I've never been trained in such a methodical and well thought-out way. As I worked out I felt as though my muscles were being stretched, and I never ached after sessions. Although it's very hard work, I was delighted to find that the programme was achievable. It was a revelation to discover that I could lift heavy weights, and actually I loved doing it.

By the end of the course, I came out of the gym feeling as happy and full of energy as when I was 16. I'd always been quite an uncontrolled eater, but after six weeks, I didn't even want to look at a chocolate. Now I only feel like eating healthy food.

Ask me

Okay, I can sense that you have some questions. Let me answer those that my clients usually ask.

Will there be results?

Does night follow day? Is the Pope a Catholic? If you follow the Bodydoctor Fitness Programme exactly, you will achieve results. My clients lose up to 6 in (15 cm) from their waists in six weeks, and, in some cases, even more. If you have it to lose, then you will drop between one and three sizes, whether a dress size or a suit size.

Do your clients do anything differently?

No! They follow exactly the same programme that you will. The only difference is that they have a trainer checking their technique at all times. In the instructions for the exercises, I list all the mistakes made by clients to help you avoid them. If you find yourself falling into these traps, just remember … Do it nice, Or do it twice! That's how I stop my clients repeating the same mistake.

Do I have to join an expensive gym?

No! You don't need to join a gym. You don't need to be wealthy to be healthy.

All the exercises in my programme require very basic equipment. The most essential piece of kit is simply a bench with an integrated foot rest, which is vital if you're to exercise in safety. The majority of gyms around the country, however (who tend to have no real interest in your needs, but are more interested in their needs) often provide benches without integrated foot

rests. For this reason, we have replicated every exercise in the workout with a Swiss stability ball (which will strengthen and support your back) and free weights, which can be cans of baked beans or bottles of water if you are starting out with the home workout.

Now this means not only can you do these exercises at home without having to join a gym at all, but if you've already joined one and it doesn't provide this basic bit of equipment, then just follow the sequence on the Home Workout pages.

Alternatively, ask your gym to buy in benches with integrated foot rests, or buy in foot rests so they can adapt their existing benches. You pay enough money for membership, so get the equipment you need!

Does it matter what time I train?

You should exercise as early in the day as possible. Your metabolic rate (that is, the number of calories you burn) is raised when you exercise. If you exercise early in the day then your metabolism is raised for longer periods. You will burn calories long after you have stopped training.

Do I have to lift heavy weights?

No! The only thing you can do with a heavy weight that you can't do with a light one is injure yourself. We've all seen those muscle men who make a lot of noise as they lift the heaviest weights in the gym. Well, bully for them. It doesn't mean that they are any fitter than those people lifting smaller weights, and often they are putting their backs at risk. And all that huffing and puffing is no use if you can't blow the house down!

It is not the weight that is important. It is the technique and number of repetitions that you can achieve with that weight. If you use a really heavy weight but can only lift it four or five times, you build up strength and size but you won't burn any fat. If you can do between 8 and 12 repetitions, you'll build muscle and burn small amounts of fat. However, if you run out of steam with a weight between 20 and 25 repetitions, you will build minimal muscle and burn maximum fat. Your dimensions will decrease, and you'll look as if you've lost a lot of weight. In reality, you may not have lost much, but this is because fat has been replaced with dense muscle – which is why I advocate the tape measure, not the scales! So working with a lighter weight achieves the best results all round.

Starting with a lighter weight also allows the muscle to get used to the movement. I believe that muscles have memories, so you need to programme them gently. If it's a graceful introduction rather than a blind date, the next time you work out, the muscles know what's coming, and they perform better. They don't recoil in shock. So, just like a first date, don't go too far the first time – get comfortable, find your level and get happy! (See the Golden Rules on page 73).

In each of your first three workouts, you should gradually increase the intensity to enable your muscles to adapt to the exercise in minimum time. This is the way to achieve maximum results. It is also the first step to working with your body, as opposed to working against it.

Now you may find that you are able to use different weights for the different exercises. This is completely normal. If you can push 15 kilos on the chest press but struggle with 4 kilos on the biceps curl, it's because your body does not have the same level of strength throughout. Some people can run for miles, for example, but are unable to lift a heavy box. But if you do push 15 kilos on the chest press and 4 kilos on the biceps curl, then it stands to reason that you could develop a great big chest and puny arms. For a uniform result, don't have too much of a gap between the weights you use. Your body can then develop proportionately.

But what happens when the weights become too easy and I can achieve 25 repetitions easily?

At this point you should progress to a heavier weight. If you choose one that still allows between 20 and 25 repetitions, it won't hinder your progress. By the way, my clients get a huge thrill when they see the weights that they use getting heavier. It shows them that their fitness levels are improving. You are no different to them. The weights will go up and you'll get that buzz. Remember, the stronger you are, the better you will feel. Doesn't everybody want to be as strong as a horse?

Ask me

Will I get big muscles?

I can't tell you how many people worry about that, but there is no risk if you follow the Bodydoctor Fitness Programme. There will be one major side effect, though: muscle weighs more than fat, so weight loss may slow as you build up lean muscles and melt down fat. But your muscles will become more defined. Many clients start to boast of six-pack stomachs, and flabby upper arms become a thing of the past.

How can I be thinner if the scales say that I have not lost much weight?

Ignore the scales! While fat may not weigh much, it does take up a large amount of space. In fact, 2½ lbs (1 kilo) of fat takes up five times the space as a similar weight of muscle. We will be replacing fat with lean muscle, and that will have a dramatic impact on your figure.

Be honest. Would you rather lose 2 stone (12.5 kilos) or go down three dress sizes? You may think that 2 stone sounds fantastic (and it is a tremendous achievement) but that may only mean losing a half-inch – a centimetre or so – all over. The Bodydoctor Fitness Programme allows you to lose all the inches you desire, while the scales may claim you have only lost a few pounds. So if you had the choice, I bet you would rather register the inch loss. After all, you can't go around with a banner saying 'I know my bum looks big in this but I have lost 2 stone'. Ignore the scales. Start to worship the tape measure – it never lies!

What do you mean by burning fat?

The exercises create heat in the muscles so that fat is used as energy. This is incredibly important, because the programme targets intra-muscular fat, which lies unseen between the muscle fibres.

When we talk about fat, most people think of subcutaneous fat that rests just below the surface of the skin. But if somebody had 35 per cent body fat, and managed to somehow shed all their subcutaneous fat, their body would not shrink by 35 per cent – they would have forgotten about the intra-muscular fat.

The best way I can describe intra-muscular fat is by imagining a joint of raw beef. This is usually plump and round, surrounded by a thick layer of fat (subcutaneous), while inside it is marbled with thin and thick layers of fat (intra-muscular). If you were to unroll the joint, scrape out all the inner layers of fat, remove the thick layer of fat and then roll it back up, you would notice that the volume of the meat dramatically falls (depending on the quantity of fat). Simply scraping off the outer layer won't achieve the same results. The human body works in exactly the same way, which is why we must address and burn fat at source for energy.

Bodydoctor

Can't I just burn fat by running around a bit?

I am not going to say that running does not burn fat because obviously it does, but frankly the best way to burn fat is through resistance exercise, like the Bodydoctor Fitness Programme, because that creates lean muscle – and lean muscle is the most efficient burner of fat. Then, when you run, your lean muscles burn more fat! Big muscles are full of fat, while small, lean muscles have powerful engines – which need a lot of fuel! And when I'm talking fuel, I mean FAT!

Cardiovascular activities, like running and swimming, exercise the heart and lungs. Your heart is a muscle that pumps blood around your body, but it doesn't use up much energy doing this – it is not a calorific exercise. Your lungs act as gas exchangers, oxygenating the blood and expelling carbon dioxide. Again, though, this is not a calorific exercise. But – and I know I'm stating the obvious here – your heart and lungs are vital. The amount of lean muscle that they feed determines your level of calorific uptake. In other words, your body's lean muscle determines the level of calories that you burn and how much energy you expend. Lots of lean muscle equals a big engine that requires lots of fuel, and as the chosen source of fuel on this programme is fat, it stands to reason that you will burn more fat.

Could you tell me a little bit more about how it works?

This book is not intended to be an encyclopaedia of exercise. It should provide you with what you need to know. No more. No less. But I know that some people enjoy the science bit so I'll let our medical man clue you in later on in the

book (see page 77). In the meantime, here is a basic bit of physiology.

Muscles contain little furnaces, known as mitochondria, where fat is burned to make energy, and adipose cells, where fat is stored. The fat furnaces and storehouses are stationed slightly apart, so fat needs to travel between the two. The transport it uses is an amino acid called L-carnitine (see also page 214). L-carnitine is produced in the body, but it is also found in foods such as offal, liver and red meat.

Therefore the amount of fat that can be burned in the muscles depends upon the level of L-carnitine in the bloodstream. If the level drops, the blood can't carry as much fat, so the muscles won't have as much fuel to burn for energy.

L-carnitine supplements are available from health shops and, subject to your doctor's approval, you might consider taking these to boost the amount of fat that your lean muscles burn at source.

Will I notice any other benefits?

What? Apart from dropping up to three sizes, doubling your fitness and losing up to a stone – around 6 kilos – in fat? Yes, there will be other benefits. You'll look good, because you only really look good when you feel good. And you'll be good: you'll have a body that can do things, rather than just wanting to be able to do things.

Muscles are the key to my programme's success, and not just because they house the furnaces that burn the fat. Muscle is king. It's your whole reason for being. It's what attracted partners to you in your prime; it's what caused your first crush. Long and lean, fit and firm,

ask me

neat and trim: muscle is everything you want to be, and everything you want in someone else. That's why muscle is so important. But it's not just the aesthetic – it's what it actually does for you. Muscle controls everything. It makes you healthy, and it's the reason you're healthy.

If your heart is pumping well and your lungs are bellowing, your vital signs are strong. You feel more alive and full of life! But when you don't exercise and use your muscles, your body gets less oxygen and somehow has to make up the deficit. So it restricts arteries, which can raise blood pressure. Arterial constriction can also increase the risk of clots and strokes, but it also makes it difficult for the cardiovascular system to respond to sudden movements. How many times have you felt dizzy after standing up quickly? That dizziness occurs because your body can't cope with a sudden increase in blood flow to the brain. Healthy muscles can help prevent this.

Most people think that osteoporosis is caused by a calcium deficiency, but it is also linked to a lack of muscular activity. Osteoporosis is a disease that occurs when bone matter fails to renew or grow. To help prevent this, you need to subject your bones to weight-bearing exercise that puts your muscles under duress. The constant resistance of having to deal with the muscle working against the bone stimulates a substance called matrix, which is used to produce new bone matter.

If you are prone to colds and sniffles, then you may not be exercising your muscles enough. Your immune system is almost totally dependent on an amino acid called glutamine, which is produced by muscle. When you exercise, your body calls upon your muscles to produce glutamine.

At Bodydoctor Fitness, that's why I don't send clients complaining that they're coming down with a cold home to put their feet up and have a hot toddy! I exercise them, although the intensity is reduced so that the immune system gets just the right boost. The correct intensity exercise boosts the immune system – it doesn't deplete it!

You can buy glutamine in supplement form from a health food shop. Unfortunately, as with some supplements, the form of glutamine won't be quite as effective as that produced by the body, because it's not created in a natural environment and won't have interacted with other vitamins and minerals. So you see, there really is no substitute for exercise! Tough!

Why do trainers always talk about heart rates?

The heart is the most important muscle in the body. It is also one of the easiest muscles to train and, as a result, has the biggest impact on your overall level of health. But it is also a fantastic indicator of just how well you are doing with your fitness programme.

The efficiency of a heart is measured by the number of times it beats in a minute as it pumps blood and oxygen around the body. Our average resting heart rate is between 60 and 80 beats per minute. However, women tend to have slightly smaller hearts than men, so their hearts actually pump a little faster to get all the blood and oxygen flowing. A whole range of factors affects our resting heart rates, from coffee (how many times has your heart raced wildly after one cup too many?) and temperature to illness, when it can increase by around 10 beats per minute. Our heart rate is even affected when we lie down. Because the heart doesn't need to fight gravity, it has less to do so the heart rate slows.

But the heart is such a clever muscle that it is possible for you to actually reduce the number of times it beats per minute when you are resting. You can make your heart work more efficiently, pumping blood and oxygen only when it is needed; then your heart won't have to work so hard. Athletes, who are exceptionally fit, usually have extremely low resting heart rates.

The maximum number of times that a man's heart can beat in one minute is theoretically 220, less his age. For a woman (remember, she has a smaller heart so a higher heart rate) it is 226 less her age. So a 40-year-old man would have, on average, a maximum heart rate of 180 beats per minute, while a 20-year-old woman would have one of 206. Every heart is individual so some people might have an unusually high maximum rate per minute.

What is your maximum heart rate?

Age	Man	Woman
20	200	206
25	195	201
30	190	196
35	185	191
40	180	186
45	175	181
50	170	176
55	165	171
60	160	166
65	155	161
70	150	156
75	145	151
80	140	146

So what should my heart rate be?

It depends upon the activity. But if you exercise at a moderate pace (which everybody does at some point during a day, either walking to the railway station or doing the weekly shop) your heart should be working at between 50 and 60 per cent of its maximum rate. But the range you're probably most interested in is the one that burns the highest percentage of fat! Generally, if you work at between 60 and 70 per cent of your maximum heart rate you'll burn fat. And it's not so hard to reach this level – walking fast or up a hill can be all that it takes. You should be feeling comfortable, not breathless. At this point you'll be using your fat resources to supply your body with energy!

But if you want to improve your overall fitness levels, you need to work your heart at between 70 and 85 per cent of its maximum rate. If you find it difficult to talk and exercise at the same time, you're probably in that zone. At this level you will be using carbohydrates as your main energy source.

The graph below shows a typical example of the type of energy used for both walking and running. Note how you burn more fat calories if you train at a lower intensity for a longer period! Remember what I said about all those men in the gym who huff and puff but don't blow the house down?

300kcal	300kcal
195 Carbohydrate	120 Carbohydrate
105 Fat	180 Fat
Running	Walking

Fat-burning: the facts

Polar, the largest and most reputable manufacturer of heart-rate monitors in the world (which has a research-and-development budget running into millions of pounds) has just launched a revolutionary range of weight management products. They monitor the heart rate, but also allow you to input your calorie intake based on the foods you eat, and calculate your calorie expenditure based on the length of time for which you exercise (see www. polar-uk.com/weightmanagement and www.bodydoctor.com).

The crucial fact here is that they recommend you train in the same zone that we at Bodydoctor Fitness advocate – namely, to burn fat you need to work at 60 to 75 per cent of your maximum heart rate! Any increase in intensity over this rate will certainly improve your aerobic fitness, but you will definitely not burn fat as efficiently. Our consistent results over a number of years backs up all their research findings.

So when one of those so-called physical experts at your gym claims that you are not working hard enough on your chosen piece of cardiovascular equipment, be comforted by the fact that some of the finest medical minds on three different continents have arrived at the same conclusion as Bodydoctor Fitness. You don't have to look like a sweaty beetroot to burn fat!

If I work out every day will I speed up the results?

Speed up the results? Isn't six weeks fast enough for you? The Bodydoctor Fitness Programme is all about developing long, lean muscle, and muscle, like every other part of the body, needs rest. Physiological changes do not take place at the time of exercise. Your strength will not miraculously improve during an exercise session. Your endurance levels will not transform over an hour or so. It is after you finish the programme that the muscles regroup, repair the damaged cells and develop. Your body needs time for that. It needs rest. So relax, put your feet up and be patient. All good things come to those who wait.

Is there any special advice I should remember?

Be realistic. If you try to change your life in a day, you'll want your old life back in a week. If you find it hard to get out of bed before eight in the morning, don't start planning to get up and go to the gym at six. Now I realize that when people finally decide to change their lives they want to change everything at once. But trust me. I've seen it so many times. They start like a whirlwind and, okay, they might manage a few early morning sessions, but by the second week they start losing the momentum. They get depressed and fall back into the old routine. You need to make time in your normal schedule for the programme and work with the resources you have. Gradually assimilate it into your routine, and soon it will fit.

Do I have to follow the nutritional advice?

Yes. But once again, be realistic. Some people are able to start both the exercise and nutritional programmes simultaneously, but others can't. They need to concentrate on one thing at a time. Well, the first thing they should concentrate on is the exercise side. It is the crux of the programme. Without exercise, all the nutrition in the world won't get you into shape – but it will dramatically improve your health, and your taste buds might get happier too. I recognize that following the nutritional advice might seem

Bodydoctor

tough if you're eating really badly. It requires you to make changes to your lifestyle, but these are minimal in relation to the immeasurable benefits you'll enjoy. But don't rush it. Over the first few days make a minor adjustment, perhaps changing what you eat for breakfast. Then over the next few days alter what you eat for lunch, and finally adjust what you have for dinner. Or slowly cut back on coffee after a certain time of the day, but gradually bring forward the time until finally you cut out coffee completely. It's very simple, isn't it? Within two weeks you will have changed your eating patterns; you will have changed your snacking patterns; and your body will swiftly respond. It's not rocket science, but it is Bodydoctor science!

How did I get started?

I know that the Bodydoctor Fitness Programme works, because it worked for me! Over the past 10 years, it has also worked for thousands of clients – most of them by mail order. I have hundreds of letters of thanks from all around the world. I have watched thousands of inches melt away from their waistlines. I have witnessed people overcome the mental struggle of actually starting their first session and then, six weeks later, sail through the programme, completely amazed at how unfit they were when they first walked through the door. Their eyes sparkle. They have more energy. They can get back into their old jeans. They look more confident. And they all follow the same programme that I developed all those years back. Remember! One size fits all – so it will definitely fit you. A fact proven by the tens of thousands of people all around the world who have used the mail order programme with equal success.

I didn't set out to discover the Holy Grail of exercise. I set out to develop a routine that

reproduced results – fast. But I also wanted a routine that I could do, achieve results and then leave alone for a couple of months. I didn't want to spend every waking hour at the gym. I had much more important things to do with my life. But I found that, as well as restoring previous fitness levels, it was also the best starter programme.

I was a fanatical football player as a child. I was always kicking a ball about, and even dreamed of becoming a professional football player. But that ended when I suffered a nasty accident to my knee at the age of 15, which left me wearing pressure bandages for a year. I had an operation that did not improve matters, and when I was finally discharged was told not to play football. Of course, I ignored the doctor's advice – and ended up having to rest for a year.

The natural fitness I had built up as a child disappeared. My speed had gone. I wanted to train, but I didn't really know how. But my innocent mind told me that, if my knee was permanently damaged, then I had to build a 'ring of steel' around it.

I believe that an injury will traumatize an area and leave a memory. At some point that memory may return, hence the saying 'my old injury is playing up.' But I didn't want my knee injury to flare up regularly and put me out of action. I wanted to develop that ring of steel so that, if it did recur, there were to be no other vulnerable areas to which it could spread.

I started going to gyms, but it was the height of Arnie Power. I watched all these lean guys getting muscle-bound bodies, with arms that didn't want to hang properly and overdeveloped legs. I just didn't see the attraction. People would walk around the gym with their arms in a sling after injuring some muscle during training as if it were an occupational hazard. The slings and crutches became badges of honour. I didn't understand it; this was supposed to be a controlled environment. These guys weren't even involved in a physical contact sport where they got nobbled, like I did.

I stopped going, and bought myself a 'Bull Worker.' It was one of those miracle gimmicks that pumps blood to your muscles when you squeeze it. It claimed that you could get a bodybuilder's physique without pumping iron! It was an isotonic and isometric exerciser, but I found that with a bit of experimentation with the machine you could get pretty good results. I started to develop different routines with the machine, as opposed to just squeezing it, and my body shape began to change. I suppose it was the first time I had ever considered working with the body.

I returned to the gym and tried new techniques but with only partial success – until somebody told me about yoga. This was 1977, way before Madonna made yoga fashionable, but it struck me that the whole theory was extremely well thought-out. There was a strict programme. Everything you did had a reason and whatever you did next had a related reason. It was sequential. Each step built upon a previous step, rather than being chucked together haphazardly.

I started to apply these ideas to what I was doing in the gym. I played around with the sequence of exercises, and really thought about how my body felt after each exertion. I looked at what the body naturally wanted to do. I began to introduce exercises that alleviated the unpleasant effects of previous ones, which was

really the precursor to my 'clean as you go' theory (see page 77). I became fitter; my body became leaner. I was able to play football again, although not at the level I had dreamed of pre-injury, and plodded on, improving my knee slowly but surely.

Then, many years later, I met an osteopath and naturopath, Philip Beach, who had a different perspective on how the body works. In two sessions he sorted out a longstanding back injury that nobody in Harley Street had been able to explain. At this point I became a sponge for knowledge. I began to look at everything from a different angle and started to apply it to my training. It was the missing link, which I combined with the knowledge gleaned from my earlier years of discovery. The Bodydoctor Fitness Programme was born.

People who know nothing of what Bodydoctor Fitness achieves call me a one-trick pony. Not so! But if you are going to be a one-trick pony, it is good to have a trick that works time after time after time. But, like any true magician, I have others up my sleeve!

How will I stay motivated?

If you really want to succeed, the results will keep you motivated. You can also read the true-life experiences of people who have followed the Bodydoctor Fitness Programme. They all highlight the speed at which their bodies reacted, the positive comments made by friends and family, and just how energized they felt. Don't just take my word for it: read these case studies of various clients, some of whom are mail-order clients and have never been close to our gym.

Bless you, my child
For you will have thinned!

When you follow this programme, I promise you that:

- **By the end of week one, you start feeling good**

- **By the end of week two, people comment on how well you look**

- **By the end of week three, you realize that you DO look good**

- **By the end of week six, you feel like a different person**

'WITHIN
6 WEEKS MARIE
HAD GONE FROM
13 STONE 7 TO
12 STONE 2,
AND TAKEN 8
INCHES OFF HER
WAIST'

CASE STUDY #1
MARIE PARCHMENT

AGE 30 **OCCUPATION** STUDENT
INCH LOSS AFTER SIX WEEKS
WAIST 8 **HIPS** 4 **CHEST** 3.875

Marie Parchment confesses to being a bit 'Billy Graham-ish' about the Bodydoctor Fitness Programme. 'I hadn't worn a belt on my jeans for years, but after three weeks I couldn't wear my jeans because they kept falling down. I had to go out and buy a belt. It was a huge psychological boost.'

'When I first spoke to David about doing the programme,' she says, 'I told him that I was a student and he told me not to spend money on coming into his gym, but just to buy the manual and do the programme by myself. Although this was good advice, I knew myself well enough to know that I wouldn't have the necessary motivation to keep up the training alone.' Weight loss was not Marie's priority when she signed up for the six-week programme. 'I just felt really unfit and unhealthy, but after every class I just felt a little bit better.'

She rigidly followed the programme, giving up alcohol and wheat, drinking 2 litres of water daily and adopting a food-combining diet. 'The nutrition part looks quite difficult, but actually it is the best thing. I am a bread and cheese girl,

but I don't want bread on its own or cheese on its own.

'I didn't want to get hung up on food, but it made me more conscious of what I was eating. I needed a decent breakfast and a proper meal after I had been to the gym.'

Within six weeks, Marie had gone from 13 stone 7 lb to 12 stone 2 lb (85.7 to 77 kilos), taken 8 in (20 cm) off her waist – 'that was just glorious' – and was nicknamed 'the shrinking one' by friends. She then carried on training by herself, taking the Bodydoctor manual to the gym. 'I have lost another stone since,' she explains, 'and I have made many changes to my life. I still go to the gym and swim, but now I do a lot more walking as well. That's something I would never have thought of doing before. The programme gave me such confidence, and physically you feel that you can do anything. Healthwise, the benefits have been massive. I feel so much better. I am more focussed with a clear head. The Bodydoctor Fitness Programme really is the best thing I ever did.'

'THE PROGRAMME COMBINES CARDIO WITH STRENGTH TRAINING, AS OPPOSED TO JUST DOING CARDIO. I FULLY BELIEVE THIS WORKS.'

CASE STUDY #2
SALLY WATERWORTH
AGE 25 **OCCUPATION** SENIOR LECTURER — SPORTS THERAPY
INCH LOSS AFTER SIX WEEKS
WAIST 3 **HIPS** 3 **CHEST** 2

Sally Waterworth is a sports scientist who admits that she cannot quite work out how the Bodydoctor Fitness Programme succeeds, but she knows that it does. Waterworth embarked on the programme after a hormone imbalance caused her to put on 3 stone in less than four months. 'A few years earlier I had been very ill, at death's door actually, after contracting shigella, a tropical disease, which basically caused my body to shut down,' she explains. The drugs to fight the infection dramatically affected her hormones. When her weight gain appeared to plateau, Sally decided to kick-start a diet with the Bodydoctor Fitness Programme. 'I had seen a television programme and read a newspaper article on it, and it looked interesting,' she continues. 'I work in sport, and everybody is lean and beautiful.

'I was already reasonably fit and did run quite a lot, but I noticed a difference within a week, really. Running certainly got easier,' she recalls.

'I have a course that I generally take. My times came down and distances went up. After 45 minutes' running I found that I could manage another hill. I didn't really expect my general fitness levels to improve so much.'

Sally didn't follow the nutrition advice — 'it didn't fit in with my lifestyle, but I ate generally more healthily' — yet she still managed to lose 7 lb (3 kilos) in six weeks. 'I lost 11 per cent of my body fat. I was really surprised.

'My parents came back from South Africa a few days after I had finished the programme, and my mother noticed a huge difference. My clothes were getting looser.'

'I STARTED AT A SIZE 12 AND 10 STONE. WITHIN 8 WEEKS, I WAS DOWN TO A SIZE 8 AND WEIGHED 8 STONE 10 POUNDS.'

CASE STUDY #3
LINDA BRAY
AGE 43 OCCUPATION HAIRDRESSER
INCH LOSS AFTER EIGHT WEEKS
WAIST 3 HIPS 3 CHEST 2 THIGH 2 LEGS 2

Linda Bray had always been fairly active, until one day she collapsed at work. 'I then slept solidly around the clock for three weeks,' she recalls. 'The doctors said 'obviously, you're exhausted, but I couldn't even string a sentence of words together. If I walked from my bedroom to the bathroom, I had to have three hours sleep to recover.' Linda had chronic fatigue syndrome.

'It is important to remember that, for chronic fatigue syndrome sufferers, a lot of the time the brain is fitter than the body. The brain wants to do something, but the body cannot comply. I remember waking early one morning and deciding to go for a walk. Within 10 minutes, my legs wouldn't walk. It took an hour to get back home. It was really a scary place to find yourself.

'I tried all sorts of detox diets. I read this book and that, searching. I saw a guy specializing in Ayurvedic Medicine but it was far too extreme for my body's needs. Nothing worked for me, but I was told that a gradual exercise programme could help. One day, flicking through a magazine, I saw an article about Sophie Dahl's transformation using the Bodydoctor Fitness Programme. Inspired, I looked through the

website, I was extremely excited by it and immediately ordered the programme.

'At first I could only do five minutes, and five repetitions. I built up very, very slowly. I had to do something every single day. I knew that I had to or I could end up permanently in a wheelchair. But I was terrified that I could set myself right back, and have absolutely no energy again. But I followed the programme to the letter.

'I began by doing three days a week, but then gradually increased the hours,' she says. Within three weeks, 'amazing things were happening, and my energy was returning.' Six weeks after starting the programme, Linda was able to return to work 'and to walk my little dog for an hour! I no longer needed my afternoon sleeps.'

Linda's doctor 'cannot believe' her patient's progress. 'I have to manage the chronic fatigue syndrome, and if I don't do the programme for a few days I can feel it building up again,' she says. 'I always do the set exercises. I was already a fairly healthy eater, but I cut out wheat and dairy, and now I no longer have asthma. That's it for life. I am on the Bodydoctor Fitness Programme.'

'I FELT REFRESHED. I HAD A LOT MORE ENERGY. THE WORKOUTS DIDN'T DRAIN ME. IN FACT, I WAS MORE TIRED WHEN I STOPPED GOING.'

CASE STUDY #4
ALAIN KEMENY
AGE 38 **OCCUPATION** RESTAURANT OWNER
INCH LOSS AFTER SIX WEEKS
WAIST 5 **HIPS** 4 **CHEST** 3
WEIGHT LOSS 6 STONE IN 8 MONTHS

When Alain Kemeny first started the Bodydoctor Fitness Programme, he was 'about 18 stone 3 lb, extremely round, very unfit' and generally ate anything he felt like. 'Clearly I wasn't happy. My waist was between 44 and 46 in, and something needed to be done,' he recalls.

It was not until his father fell ill, that something was done. 'One of the surgeons commented that the risk to my father would have been lower if he had not been so overweight. It stuck in my mind, and I decided to act.'

He embarked on the programme, combining it with changes to his lifestyle. 'I kept away from fat, dramatically cut down dairy and starch and cut out coffee and sugar completely. I also drank a lot of water, and started walking everywhere,' he says. 'I took it slowly. I didn't think everything would change overnight.'

But it did. Within one week, Alain felt better. Within three weeks, he noticed that his muscles were more defined 'where the fat used to be. At four weeks, I noticed quite clearly that my trousers were getting looser – that's all the time it took.' When he finished the six-week programme, Alain bought trousers two sizes smaller than his usual size. 'You notice some improvements very quickly, and that made me want to continue the process.'

Eight months after Alain began the programme, his weight had dropped to just under 12 stone – a loss of just over 6 stone (76 kilos). 'My waist was down to 32 in. There had been some periods where my weight seemed to stabilize, but I just worked through them.'

He adds: 'I felt refreshed. I had a lot more energy. The workouts didn't drain me. In fact, I was more tired when I stopped going. There are elements of discomfort with some exercises, but anybody can do this. It is certainly not difficult.'

'WITHIN 6 WEEKS I HAD LOST A COUPLE OF DRESS SIZES, AND IN 12 WEEKS I HAD LOST ABOUT 4.' EVEN HER SHOE SIZE ALTERED.

CASE STUDY #5
RACHEL DAVIS
AGE 31 **OCCUPATION** TRAINEE SOLICITOR
INCH LOSS AFTER SIX WEEKS
WAIST 8 **HIPS** 4 **THIGH** 3.5 **CHEST** 1
WEIGHT LOSS 1 **STONE** 6 **POUNDS**

When Rachel Davis determined to get in shape for her forthcoming wedding, she was adamant that a slimming group was not for her. 'I needed a diet and exercise programme. I actually wanted to change my body shape and sustain it. I wanted more muscle and less fat,' she explains. 'I knew that I could go on a diet and lose weight, but I worried that I'd put it back on as soon as I'd finished it.'

Rachel also decided against signing up for exercise classes. 'I wasn't terribly active. I had asthma, I weighed a lot more than I should, and my lifestyle was sedentary,' she says. 'It would have been quite challenging for me to go to a gym and jump straight in. I needed something that I could work at, rather than being forced to stand at the front of an aerobic class and puff and pant with everybody watching.'

She opted for the Bodydoctor Fitness Programme. 'I followed it exactly, doing the exercises in the right order. I just decided that there was no point in doing it if I wasn't going to do it properly.' She also followed the nutritional advice. 'After the first few days of not eating refined sugar, I stopped wanting it,' she says. Although Davis did not restrict portion sizes, she found that 'trying

to chew each mouthful fifty times meant that I didn't eat loads.'

Davis started with low weights to achieve between 20 or 25 repetitions. 'I didn't want to overdo it and have an asthma attack, but I soon found that I was able to deal with bigger and bigger weights,' she recalls, 'and that was a huge thrill. My energy levels improved, as did my physical strength and stamina,' she says. 'Within six weeks I had lost a couple of dress sizes, and in 12 weeks I had lost about four.' Even her shoe size altered. 'I must admit I was a bit shy about going to the gym and tried to keep it quiet at first, but when people kept coming up to me asking me what I had done to lose weight I had to confess! The best thing was that my asthma seemed to disappear. It's an incredible feeling to regain your lung capacity after years of feeling like you're dependant on your inhaler.'

'Losing weight became expensive because I had to throw out clothes and buy new ones,' she says. 'Now it is really nice to be able to wear the clothes that I want, say if I see something in a magazine, and not even think about being able to get it in my size.' And for her wedding? 'I wore the dress I had always wanted.'

'WITHIN 4 WEEKS ALMOST ALL MY EXCESS WEIGHT CAME OFF. I WOULD SAY IT WAS A GOOD STONE AND A HALF.'

CASE STUDY #6
ANT McPARTLIN
AGE 27 **OCCUPATION** TELEVISION PRESENTER
INCH LOSS AFTER SIX WEEKS
WAIST 4 **HIPS** 2 **CHEST** 1

Ant McPartlin might seem self-assured in front of the cameras, but he admits, 'when I feel a little bit bigger, I don't feel very confident. And you are reminded of that insecurity on a weekly basis when you do a live television series'.

So before the first *Pop Idol* series hit the screens (and long before Gareth Gates and Will Young became household names), Ant and his best friend Dec signed up for the Bodydoctor. 'I never really trained properly before,' he says. 'I went to the gym and was fairly active. I could run around a bit, but my strength wasn't great. I wanted to be fitter and feel better.'

Ant adds: 'I wanted to tone up, but I didn't want to get loads of muscles. I just wanted to be confident when my shirt came off!'

For six weeks he stuck rigidly to the programme, adopting the nutrition plan as well. 'You find what food suits you,' he says. 'I used to get lethargic after carbohydrates, so I now eat much more protein. I just don't feel as stuffed and bloated afterwards.' The first real session was 'a massive uphill struggle and six weeks seemed a lifetime ahead' but within four weeks 'almost all my excess weight came off. I would say it was a good stone and a half. I was getting into old jeans and I had to buy myself new shirts. The size went down from a large to a medium.'

There was another unexpected benefit. 'I used to have a bad back, and I found the ab-flow really hurt my lower back at first. So we wouldn't do a lot, but then we added a little bit more,' says Ant. 'It turned out that I had no real stomach strength and my back was being forced to compensate. Now my stomach is stronger and I have no back troubles. I didn't think that I would get anything like that out of the programme.'

Ant, who describes his lifestyle as 'hectic,' says he has learned to incorporate the programme into his schedule. 'I am much more aware of my fitness levels,' he says. 'You go to the gym and you feel better, but when you stop going you start feeling run down. You hear of all those ridiculous diets, like only eat green food for six days, but, at the end of the day, you have got to exercise. It is the easiest and simplest way to lose weight and get fit.'

'PEOPLE TOLD ME I HAD LOST A LOT OF WEIGHT, AND MY EYES WERE MORE SPARKLY. I JUST LOOKED FRESH. I WAS SLEEPING BETTER.'

CASE STUDY #7
DEC DONNELLY
AGE 27 OCCUPATION TELEVISION PRESENTER
INCH LOSS AFTER SIX WEEKS
WAIST 3 HIPS 1 CHEST 1

Dec Donnelly was delighted by the reaction of his tailor when he went along for a suit fitting. 'I had lost 3 in off my waist. My tailor said, "My God, what has happened?" I told him that I'd been to the Bodydoctor. I was getting into jeans I hadn't worn for years.'

Dec's waist was not the only visible difference. 'People told me I had lost a lot of weight, and my eyes were more sparkly. I just looked fresh. I was sleeping better,' he says. Even the football team he played with every weekend noticed a change. 'I used to be exhausted during the last 10 to 15 minutes, but now I could have kept going for another half an hour,' Dec explains. 'I was getting forward much more, and getting into the box.'

Like so many people, Dec used to promise himself every New Year that he would get fit. 'Every January I would go in and run for half an hour on a treadmill because that seemed a popular thing to do, then I'd lift some weights

and do a few sit ups. The Bodydoctor Fitness Programme actually taught me how to exercise.'

He adds: 'I think David thought we were a bit soft. I was not hugely obese, but I was squidgy and a bit soft. I knew that I wanted toned muscles, because I had heard that phrase on the telly. With the Bodydoctor, I actually burned fat and toned muscle. I don't know how I did it, but it certainly happened.' Dec is such a fan that he has encouraged both brothers and his girlfriend to have a go.

Dec stuck rigidly to the nutrition plan for the first six weeks 'although I still partook of alcohol,' but he has since adapted it. 'I don't drink as much beer as I used to. I drink more wine, and I kind of stay off bread,' he explains. 'You have to be able to have a life as well. But this programme has taught me how to exercise. It is the best thing, fitness-wise, that I have ever done.'

'THE BOTTOM LINE IS: IT WORKS. IT CLAIMS TO GET YOU BACK INTO PRE-PREGNANCY JEANS WITHIN 6 WEEKS — BY GOD, IT DOES!'

CASE STUDY #8
CLAIRE HARRISON

AGE 31 **OCCUPATION** RUNS A BUSINESS FROM HOME
INCH LOSS AFTER SIX WEEKS
WAIST 2 **HIPS** 2 **CHEST** 1

Claire Harrison had never had a problem with her weight, but her figure took rather a battering when she had four children in just three years. 'I had my first child in 1999 when I put on 4 stone; twins in 2001, which meant I put on 6 stone; and another child, Ben, in July 2002, when I gained 3 stone,' she says. 'I put the weight on with the first pregnancy, and never really lost it.'

She had unsuccessfully tried many other diets before she started the Bodydoctor Fitness Programme. 'I wanted to lose weight, get my shape back to where it had been, particularly my stomach, and to retain my pre-children levels of fitness.'

Claire did not follow the nutrition advice, but rigidly adhered to the exercise programme. 'I worked really hard in the sessions, and within two or three weeks I was noticing a difference. My husband started to comment on my figure, as did my friends,' she says. 'Every bit of excess weight was gone after six weeks. I lost at least one-and-a-half dress sizes, but my shape also changed. The muscles in my legs were really apparent, and my husband even pointed out that I was getting a six-pack! I am even able to wear short-sleeved tops now.'

At the end of the programme, Claire found that her fitness levels were back to where they were before she had her four sons. 'In fact, now I am easily fitter than I was,' she admits. 'The evidence is there, and the results are much better than I ever expected.'

Claire now combines the Bodydoctor workout with Pilates. 'I genuinely do believe that this is the fastest way to shed weight and get fit,' she says. 'The bottom line is that you read about the programme and its claim to get you back into pre-pregnancy jeans within six weeks, and you wonder. By God, it works!'

'MY DIABETES BECAME MORE STABLE THAN BEFORE. MY SUGAR LEVELS SEEMED TO SORT THEMSELVES OUT.'

CASE STUDY #9
DIGBY LOCK
AGE 29 **OCCUPATION** IT SPECIALIST
INCH LOSS AFTER SIX WEEKS
WAIST 3 **HIPS** 1 **CHEST** 2

Digby Lock is typical of many people. Extremely active at university, enjoying cross-country running, tennis and rugby, Digby now spends his days sitting in front of a computer. 'I would definitely say my lifestyle is sedentary now,' he admits. 'I'm tall and, before I started the programme, I wasn't really overweight, but there is a wide range of acceptable weights and I was up near the top of that.'

Digby chose the Bodydoctor Fitness Programme because 'it seemed to deliver what it promised in a reasonable period of time,' he says. 'I quite liked the fact that the thinking was taken out of my hands. Even if it looked like nothing was happening, I was assured that if I persisted then there would be results.'

Digby did not notice any weight loss but he 'noticed fat loss within four weeks, perhaps even sooner, but strengthwise I noticed it much sooner. I was visibly stronger. When I started the programme, I couldn't do very much for very long. Things seemed impossible, but then suddenly I was able to do it.'

By the end of six weeks, Digby was pulling his belt a further three notches tighter. 'Generally I felt so much healthier. I seemed to have so much more energy,' he says.

Digby is a diabetic. He did not want to cut out carbohydrates, although nutritionists recommend that diabetics limit carbohydrate intake. Digby adds: 'I did make sure that I was eating reasonably healthily. It is much easier to eat unhealthy things and to miss out breakfast.'

Digby also experienced an unexpected benefit from the Bodydoctor Fitness Programme. 'My diabetes became more stable than before,' he says. 'My sugar levels seemed to sort themselves out. When I did have to miss a meal, the effect was nowhere near as dramatic as it had been in the past. I can now get away with some vices that would normally have sent my sugar levels right up.'

'CONSIDERING I WAS DOING IT AT A SLOWER PACE TO EVERYBODY ELSE, I WAS SHOCKED THAT 4" CAME OFF MY WAIST IN 6 WEEKS.'

CASE STUDY #10
NANCY PAGANI

AGE 33 **OCCUPATION** DESIGNER AND MOTHER
INCH LOSS AFTER SIX WEEKS
WAIST 4 **HIPS** 3 **CHEST** 3

Nancy Pagani spent days unpacking boxes after she moved house. While other people might get depressed at such an activity, Pagani actually revelled in it, because it would have been impossible before she completed the Bodydoctor Fitness Programme.

Nancy suffered three prolapsed discs when she was 18. 'I was getting out of a car, and suddenly I was in absolute agony. I had to lie down for a week.' The injury was never resolved and regularly put her out of action. 'Once a year I would end up spending seven weeks in bed,' she says. Exercise was impossible.

Her desire for a baby sent her to an osteopath. 'He put me on the straight and narrow, and pregnancy made my back malleable. He was able to repair parts of my back.' The osteopath also suggested exercise to aid the recovery process.

'I almost cried the first time I went to the Bodydoctor, because I was so scared that I

would be laid up,' she admits. 'But it just seemed the right way. I had to find my level in every exercise.'

In her first session, Nancy managed just 20 ab curls – 'I was hopeless' – but six weeks later, she was doing 140. 'There were a fair amount of exercises that I was not able to do, such as squats or lunges, but I was shown how to do the same exercises on a machine, which protected my back because I was lying down.'

By the end of the programme 'I was so much healthier. I felt fit and strong. Everybody noticed. I lost a little bit of weight and one third of my body fat. It was absolutely amazing.' She adds: 'Considering I was doing it all at a slower pace to everybody else, I was shocked that I took 4 in off my waist in six weeks.

'Honest to God, my back didn't give way or hurt once. I learned that there is a way for me to do exercise. I would recommend that everybody tries it.'

'I FOOLED THE ENTIRE AGENCY. I WAS EVEN OFFERED A JOB AT STRINGFELLOW'S AS A TABLE DANCER AND THOSE GIRLS ARE REALLY FIT.'

CASE STUDY #11
LISA BRINKWORTH
AGE 31 OCCUPATION JOURNALIST/TV PRODUCER
INCH LOSS AFTER SIX WEEKS
WAIST 3 HIPS 3 CHEST 2

Lisa Brinkworth always hated exercise. She was the girl at school who found excuses to miss her PE lessons. Not that she needed to sweat at the gym, though – Lisa was a trim size 10, who never considered herself overweight until five years ago when she was asked to go undercover as a model for the television series *McIntyre Undercover*.

Lisa explains: 'I had to get myself signed on the books of a model agency in Milan. I did my research, and realized that I had to be a size 8 to achieve that.'

She needed results fast, and turned to the Bodydoctor. 'My body completely changed shape as a result. I was slim but I had never had a small waist, yet soon I lost a couple of inches off it. My shape was much more defined, and for the first time in my life I had a completely flat stomach.'

She adds: 'My arms toned up, my shoulders looked better. People started commenting on my figure.' The transformation worked. The BBC mocked up a portfolio of photographs, and Lisa was signed up as an older model with a leading agency (which cannot be named for legal reasons). 'I fooled the entire agency into thinking I was a model. I had a mini-disc recorder

strapped to my hip, and the only negative comment I ever had was that my left hip was slightly bigger than my right one.'

After the agency discovered the truth, its head claimed that they never really thought that Lisa was a model. 'They became really uncomplimentary,' she says. 'But I truly fooled them. I lived in the models' residence with the other models, and they were very interested in what I was doing in the gym.'

'Each night I had to view my tapes, and listen back over the day's activities. I would work into the early hours, and got very little sleep. I really wouldn't have survived without exercising. I felt so much fitter. I would wake up with little difficulty.'

Even when Lisa stopped training regularly for a year, she retained her longed-for waist. And when she had to get back into perfect shape to go undercover as a lap dancer, Lisa returned to the Bodydoctor. 'I am a firm believer in muscles having a memory,' she says. 'The results were really quick.' The assignment was a success. 'I was even offered a job at Stringfellow's as a table dancer, and those girls are really fit.'

IN 10 WEEKS, KAY SHED 6" OFF HER WAIST. IN 4 MONTHS SHE LOST 2¾ STONE. 'I NEVER WANT TO FEEL THAT UNFIT AND UNHAPPY AGAIN.'

CASE STUDY #12
KAY ACOTT

AGE 34 **OCCUPATION** CLIENT DIRECTOR
INCH LOSS AFTER SIX WEEKS
WAIST 3 **HIPS** 4 **CHEST** 4

Kay Acott had reached rock bottom before she started the Bodydoctor Fitness Programme. She was unfit and overweight – a combination of a new baby and a job that required entertaining clients – and, after seeing a photograph of herself on holiday, quite depressed. She had tried various forms of exercise and diets, but just couldn't find anything that made a difference.

Kay did the exercise programme three times a week, but adapted the nutritional side to fit in with her lifestyle. 'I generally tried not to eat protein and carbohydrate at the same time and cut out alcohol between Monday and Thursday, when I was really good. But on Friday and Saturday all bets were off. I just felt that I had worked all week and I really needed a couple of glasses of wine. On Sunday I just tried to get back into it,' she explains. 'I cut out dairy, although I did keep eating cheese. I also cut out wheat on David's advice, and felt so much better.

For Kay, the programme took a little while to kick in. 'My fitness levels really improved within about four weeks and I was feeling a difference in terms of muscle tone,' she says, 'but I wasn't really losing weight or inches at that point. That's probably a

result of not abstaining from all things delicious, such as cheese and wine. However, I stayed focussed on the goal I had set myself, which was to get into (and look good in) a pair of fitted jeans and a fitted white shirt, instead of my husband's jeans and an oversized baggy white shirt.'

David encouraged Kay to be patient and persevere. 'David kept telling me that my metabolism would be speeding up and that my increased muscle tone would start to have an impact on burning up fat. I was so determined to give the programme a chance,' she says, 'I didn't want to go back to the way I had been feeling. Then suddenly it kicked in. It was incredible. I started losing so much weight that people kept asking me if I was really eating. They were shocked. I transformed from an absolute pear shape.'

'The programme has been absolutely fantastic for me. Getting into an exercise routine that is hugely enjoyable, and adopting a style of eating that does not involve dieting, has allowed me to feel in control of my body again. I shall never forget the delicious feeling of going into Gap and finding that a size-13 pair of 'long and lean' hipster jeans actually fitted me.'

'IF I HADN'T STARTED THE PROGRAMME, THEN I REALLY BELIEVE THAT I WOULD HAVE HAD A HEART ATTACK IN MY THIRTIES.'

CASE STUDY #13
PAUL ADAMS
AGE 31 **OCCUPATION** REPRESENTATIVE OF RECORD PRODUCERS
INCH LOSS AFTER SIX WEEKS
WAIST 6 **CHEST** 5
WEIGHT LOSS 6 **STONE IN** 8 **MONTHS**

When Paul Adams first turned up at the Bodydoctor Gym, David Marshall seriously worried that Paul might have a heart attack. 'He put me on the Stairmaster, with just two dots lit up, and I could only manage a minute and a half. I thought I was going to die,' recalls Paul. 'I weighed in at 24½ stone. David told me later that he was really concerned.'

But David didn't confide these fears to Paul. Instead he was full of encouragement. 'A week after I joined, this guy, who had only started two or three weeks before me, lost a stone. David told me that I would achieve even more. One week later I lost my first stone.'

Paul followed all the nutritional advice. 'I cut out refined sugar. Even now, years later, I still don't touch it. I also used to drink two or three pints a night, watching bands, and I stopped drinking for two six-week sessions.' Paul was also taught that 'it's not about the scales. I would be building muscle, which weighs heavier than fat, so I should be more interested in the tape measure.'

The first week, Paul 'felt like hell.' He adds: 'David told me that it wasn't about the weights

you lift, but it was about the repetitions. It was about your body entering a fat-burning phase. I had seen various trainers before, but nobody had ever told me that. It made sense.'

Last year, Paul moved to New York and enrolled in a gym. 'The trainer told me that it was all about the biggest weights, and when I managed to lift them five times, he told me that I was doing great. I was absolutely exhausted and all I could think was, "this goes against everything I ever learned with David." I dumped the trainer, and started back on the Bodydoctor Fitness Programme.' He adds: 'The bottom line is that the body responds well to the programme. David told me what it would do for me, and it did it.'

Paul admits that he 'tried to exceed all expectations; when I was told to do one more repetition, I would do five.' At the end of six weeks, he stood on the Stairmaster and 'with all the dots lit up' managed 10 full minutes. 'I don't think even David believed I would be able to do that.' But the biggest buzz for Paul came three weeks after he started the programme, when a friend said, 'Big fella, are you losing weight?' 'That was brilliant,' Paul reflects. Paul eventually lost six stone.

'I JUST FOUND MYSELF TEN TIMES FITTER. IT HAS BEEN AN EYE-OPENING EXPERIENCE.'

CASE STUDY #14
ALEX FRICK

AGE 52 **OCCUPATION** PRIVATE INVESTOR
INCH LOSS AFTER SIX WEEKS
WAIST 2 **HIPS** 1 **CHEST** 1

Alex Frick had always viewed himself as an active man. He cycled and spent between 30 and 60 days a year skiing. So he was a little bemused when his wife bought him a six-week programme with Bodydoctor Fitness as his Christmas present. 'I was scratching my head,' he admits, particularly as it turned out that it was he – not his wife who was actually paying for it!

'I really enjoyed the first session. They had a very precise and specific approach to fitness. I was the classic example of a guy who went to the gym and huffed and puffed without accomplishing his objectives. I learned to do everything a different way.'

Alex's passion is skiing, particularly heli-skiing, but he was getting older, and admits that, as a result, on the first day of a skiing trip 'I couldn't just put on my skis and spend the whole day skiing. I couldn't ski the first afternoon.'

The top lifts for heli-skiing can be 5000 m (16,405 ft) high, and Alex says that skiers need to be 'pretty fit to deal with the high altitudes.' He had an Indian heli-skiing trip planned for a month after his first session at Bodydoctor Fitness. 'The first day went like a breeze,' he recalls. 'I was the oldest guy in a group of four, the others were all in their twenties and thirties, but I was the only one who could go on all day.'

At the end of the week, the organizers count how many vertical feet the skiers have travelled – reflecting the number of jumps. Alex's trip had been interrupted by a two-day bout of dysentery, yet he recorded the most vertical feet. 'I just found myself ten times fitter. It has been an eye-opening experience.'

Alex, who did not follow the nutrition plan but claims he always eats healthily, actually put on weight as he built new muscles 'but my body fat fell a few per cent.'

The programme has also helped Alex in unexpected ways. 'I race cars and you need to be physically fit to do that. The cockpit is extremely hot, you swing from side to side and a lot of physical effort is involved. I was involved in a bit of a wreck at the weekend, but I was actually fine.'

'I AM CONVINCED THAT OTHERS WITH DIABETES, WHETHER INSULIN DEPENDENT OR NOT, WOULD BENEFIT FROM THE PROGRAMME.'

CASE STUDY #15
RENATA DRINKWATER
AGE 47 OCCUPATION INT. MANAGEMENT CONSULTANT (LEISURE & TOURISM)
INCH LOSS AFTER SIX WEEKS
WAIST 2.5 HIPS 2 CHEST 1

Renata Drinkwater had an active lifestyle and both a personal and professional interest in health and fitness, but felt she wasn't really improving her fitness levels.

Things only started to change when Renata read about the Bodydoctor Fitness Programme in a magazine. 'I was immediately struck by the fact that although David's approach looked unorthodox, it was producing truly fantastic – and very speedy – results. I was also impressed by David's idea of working opposing muscle groups sequentially to avoid the need for extensive stretching after the programme, so making the best use of time. Time was important to me – I wanted to get fitter, stronger and help control my diabetes as quickly as possible!' she admits.

Renata had developed insulin-dependent diabetes several years earlier and knew exercise would be crucial in controlling this serious condition. She also followed a low-carbohydrate diet. Though not recommended for people with Type I diabetes, she found it 'particularly effective.' Combining this with the programme, the results were sensational.

Within two or three weeks, Renata noticed results. 'I lost a few pounds. I felt better and looked better. Also, I didn't experience the aches and pains that accompanied other fitness programmes I'd tried.' Renata also felt better equipped to cope with the stress of her job, 'I just felt that I could deal with all those stresses,' she says. She even found that the programme speeded up her recovery period after major surgery.

But it was the dramatic benefits to her Type I diabetes that stunned Renata, who is also a member of the advisory council for Diabetes UK. 'My average blood glucose levels dropped around 10 per cent and I was able to reduce the amount of insulin I was taking by about 15 per cent,' she says. 'I can only attribute this to the programme as I had made no other changes to my regime, and had been continuing to follow a low-carbohydrate diet as before.' Renata also discovered more benefits of the programme when she underwent hospital tests. 'The tests have shown that my long-term blood glucose control is on target and that other key indicators, such as blood pressure, are good. Getting fitter could mean being able to reduce – and in some cases even stop – medication, with less chance of serious diabetic damage to the eyes, kidneys, nerves, heart and major arteries.'

'AFTER 3 WEEKS, I FOUND THAT MY CLOTHES WERE BECOMING LOOSER, AFTER 6 WEEKS I HAD DROPPED 3 DRESS SIZES.'

CASE STUDY #16
EVA INZANI
AGE 38 **OCCUPATION** COFFEE IMPORTER
INCH LOSS AFTER SIX WEEKS
WAIST 5 **HIPS** 4 **THIGHS** 3 **CHEST** 2 **SHOULDERS** 2

Eva Inzani had not exercised since university and had no real inclination to. She had been a size 10 for years and ate whatever she liked. But when Eva set up her own business, things changed. 'I found that my weight was going up and my clothes were becoming much tighter, but I was still very busy with my new business and I ignored the problem.'

It was the onset of summer and the thought of wearing short sleeves, slinky clothes and bikinis galvanized her into action. 'I decided to find a quick solution,' she states, 'but I had never been to a gym before and didn't want to go somewhere really impersonal.'

Eva saw an article in *Marie Claire* magazine, which showed the results of the Bodydoctor Programme. 'I was inspired that the results were so definite and quick,' she recalls. Eva was also looking for a fitness programme for her sister, Natasha, who was both a size 6 and 6 ft tall. 'After two seasons snowboarding, Natasha had returned to the UK really thin and she had lost far too much weight. Natasha has always been slim and she had tried hundreds of ways to gain weight – including powder drink supplements and eating copious amounts of fatty foods,' says Eva.

But Natasha's fast metabolism meant that she did not put weight on.

'I rang the Bodydoctor and explained to David that I needed to lose weight and Natasha needed to put weight on,' she recalls. 'I asked David if this was possible. He explained that we could both achieve our objectives by following the programme, because it gets the body back into its natural state of balance.

'I was slightly sceptical that it would work for Natasha, but I was keen to try any possible solution. We both joined at exactly the same time,' says Eva. She followed the nutrition programme religiously – dropping alcohol, wheat and dairy from her diet. People began complimenting her on how healthy she looked. 'I had stacks more energy and a brighter complexion.'

Eva had worried that working with weights would make her develop muscles. 'Instead, I found that my arms and legs were much slimmer and toned – almost flattened – and that my thighs had permanently shrunk by three inches.' In contrast, Natasha actually put weight on in all the right places. 'She went up two sizes but looked very healthy and toned,' says Eva.

'DAVID TALKS A LANGUAGE EVERYONE UNDERSTANDS. HE MANAGED TO GET THE TEAM WORKING REALLY HARD.'

CASE STUDY #17
HARRY REDKNAPP
AGE 56 **OCCUPATION** FOOTBALL MANAGER, PORTSMOUTH
NO MEASUREMENTS TAKEN

David Marshall is a lifelong West Ham fan, so it is perhaps not surprising that he offered his services to Harry Redknapp when he was manager of the team. 'The lads needed strengthening,' recalls Harry. 'They lacked upper body strength. It wasn't the case that they needed to build muscle mass, but they did need to develop strength. David knew how to do that. He knew how to get the best out of the players and coincidentally during his time there the team climbed from twentieth position to sixth.'

Harry felt that David 'talks a language everybody understands. He managed to get the team working hard, and really improved their level of fitness. They felt much better.'

David did not work with all the players, but trained an impressive selection, including Rio Ferdinand, Joe Cole, Trevor Sinclair and Frank Lampard. 'All of them played for England,' recalls Harry. 'I certainly think that David improved their fitness levels a great deal.'

But Harry didn't try out the Bodydoctor Fitness Programme. 'No, I didn't. I think I am too old. However, Roger Cross — who was my first team coach and is still at West Ham — said that David was absolutely in a different class and it was the best training he'd come across in 25 years. I'd recommend him without a doubt. He really is excellent.'

'I AM STRONGER ON THE PITCH AND HAVE NOTICED A GREAT IMPROVEMENT IN MY PLAYING SINCE TRAINING WITH HIM.'

CASE STUDY #18
RIO FERDINAND
AGE 24 **OCCUPATION** PROFESSIONAL FOOTBALLER
NO MEASUREMENTS TAKEN

Rio Ferdinand is full of praise for David's methods. He started training with David six weeks before establishing himself as an England regular. 'I was fit before, but David took me to the next level,' he says. 'I am stronger on the pitch and have noticed a great improvement in my playing since training with him. It had definitely enhanced my football and if it makes you look better in the mirror – which it has – then that's an added bonus.'

Rio was 20 when he first started training with David Marshall. He was one of the younger members of West Ham and, like so many other football players, had neglected the need for weight training. 'I always thought that if you did weight training, then you would put on weight and wouldn't be able to run,' he recalls. 'I thought I would get too bulky. But I was at a stage in my career when I really needed to add to my game.'

When David arrived to spice up the training programme for the team, Rio was impressed. 'He was very enthusiastic. He came and chatted and he seemed knowledgeable and experienced. He pointed out that sprinters do weight training,

and that they're not all big and muscular. I just didn't know how to train with weights.'
Rio began to adopt the Bodydoctor Fitness Programme. 'After four to five weeks, I felt a lot stronger. I felt different,' he recalls. 'I was always able to run for long periods, but I can now produce some explosive bursts. It made a definite difference.'

'Trevor Sinclair, Jermaine Defoe and I – we all benefited from training with David. We incorporated his sessions into our own workouts. It enhanced us as footballers – and we have all played for England at some level!'

Now at Manchester United, Rio still does the programme two or three times a week. 'It obviously depends on the games. Everybody has their own routine to do, and I now have mine!'

Since training with David, Ferdinand has become an England regular and the bedrock of their defence, while other players who followed the programme – such as Trevor Sinclair, Michael Carrick, Joe Cole and Frank Lampard – are now also regulars in the squad.

'THE PROGRAMME IS AN INVALUABLE TOOL FOR MODERN LIFE. IT IS A GREAT DEFENCE AGAINST THE RISE OF MODERN DISEASE — OBESITY.'

CASE STUDY #19
DR KATE PICKERING
AGE 41 OCCUPATION GENERAL PRACTITIONER IN GLASGOW
NO MEASUREMENTS TAKEN

Kate Pickering was an early convert to Bodydoctor Fitness. About ten years ago she read about the programme and sent off for a booklet. 'I'm 5 ft 10 in and have had three children, so I feel best between 10½–11½ stone. Whenever I go up to 12½ stone, I follow the programme and within 8 to 10 weeks I find that I have lost a stone and toned up quite a bit. So when my patients ask me what I do, I just say do it yourself.'

She adds: 'I started to lend the programme to my patients. Going to the gym is all very well for motivated people but I had working mothers coming to see me, who just had no free time. They needed something that was just not gym based. Also, it's not terribly complex, which appeals to my patients.'

Dr Pickering was also attracted to the nutrition side. 'We eat far too much carbohydrate, which is responsible for the explosion in Type II diabetes, heart disease and polycystic ovaries. We need to change our diets to eat more protein and less carbohydrate, which is what I am saying to my patients. David has definitely had the right idea all along.'

Recently, Dr Pickering advised a patient with polycystic ovaries to adopt the programme. 'It made a massive difference. She is now pregnant, and she was infertile before.' Of course, Dr Pickering knows that one patient may not be typical of others, but she adds: 'If a woman comes to me who is 3 stone overweight and excessively hairy, then I would tell her to lose the weight first to stabilize her blood sugars and get her hormones into balance.'

Dr Pickering is currently using the programme on a cross-section of patients suffering from Type II diabetes. 'I am really excited. The programme is an invaluable tool for modern life. It is a great defence against the rise of modern disease – obesity – which can lead to Type II diabetes and heart disease.

'DAVID WAS VERY STRICT ABOUT DOING THE EXERCISES PROPERLY. HE IS QUITE PARTICULAR ABOUT THE SAFETY ASPECT.'

CASE STUDY #20
NICKY CLARKE
AGE 46 **OCCUPATION** CELEBRITY HAIRDRESSER
INCH LOSS AFTER SIX WEEKS
WAIST 3 **HIPS** 2 **CHEST** 1 **SHOULDERS** 1

Nicky Clarke has known David Marshall for many years. He first started training with him when Marshall had a gym in his house. 'I was fairly gym orientated,' he recalls. 'I had read all about different types of exercise, so David wasn't explaining his programme to somebody who didn't understand.'

The programme has evolved over the years. 'He had perfected a simple yet sophisticated approach. He applies the same method to everybody, but just changes the intensity and weights. There are a lot of similarities between the way I work when I cut hair. I use the same method of sectioning for different types of hairstyles. A lot of people found that incredibly difficult to grasp.'

'David was unconventional, because he said "do one set of 25 repetitions," when everyone else was saying, "do three sets." I did think it went against everything I had read. He insisted on no real rest period, not hitting the same muscle part often, and equalizing each muscle with an opposite number. But there was no kind of pain threshold 24 hours later.'

Nicky began exercising 'not because I wanted to lose weight, but if I don't do anything then I can quite easily add three quarters of a stone and it is not a nice three quarters of a stone!' But he wanted to 'lose a percentage of body fat.'

'David was very strict about doing the exercises properly. He would drop my weights down in order to make sure that I did them correctly. He is quite particular about the safety aspect and the programme is obviously well thought out.'

Nicky got results 'relatively immediately.' Today he finds it difficult to pop into David's Primrose Hill gym, but takes his manual along to his local one. 'I am quite strict about doing it two or three times a week. Once I saw somebody who was quite clearly following David's programme at my local gym. If I don't have time for a full work-out, then I will do all the exercises without the aerobics. I can do them in half an hour – I know it will be a tough half-hour, but that I will be in fairly decent shape afterwards.'

'I WAS SO IMPRESSED, THAT I JOINED THE COMPANY! IT WAS A COMPLETE INSPIRATION TO ME.'

CASE STUDY #21
STEVE MARSHALL

AGE 31 **OCCUPATION** TRAINER AT BODYDOCTOR FITNESS
INCH LOSS AFTER SIX WEEKS
WAIST 5 **HIPS** 4 **THIGH** 3 **CHEST** 5 **SHOULDERS** 3

Steve Marshall lost 5 stone over five months on the Bodydoctor Fitness Programme. He was so impressed that he joined the company. And no, he is not related to David Marshall!

Steve was at college studying Sports Therapy when his mother started training with the Bodydoctor. 'I just wanted to meet him and see what it was all about.' Steve, who had once played rugby for Wasps and had been in the reserve England Under-21 squad, had piled on the pounds when he gave up the game. 'I had not exercised in about 18 months and was eating the same amount of food as I had when playing rugby,' he admits. 'I sat down and had a chat with David and agreed to start doing the programme. I did it once a week with him, and twice a week on my own.'

Steve had a serious knee injury that has required 19 operations to date. It prevented him doing lunges, and he could only do squats with a low weight. He also did extra cardio work. 'I pushed myself,' he recalls. 'I know how hard you can push yourself when you want to.

'Because of my rugby background, I had lived off carbohydrates all my life. I cut those out

pretty fast. I didn't touch gluten, bread, pasta or dairy and I introduced portion control. I also didn't drink alcohol,' he recalls. Two stone fell off within seven weeks. 'After two months, friends were saying, "you look like you have lost a lot of weight." It was just falling off. And I was sleeping a hell of a lot better. I would wake up and get up. I had always been someone who hit the snooze button. My posture improved.' He was also surprised to discover that the programme did not aggravate his knee injury. Steve admits that his weight loss stabilized after two months – he hit a plateau – but then 'after another month, a load more came off.'

As a rugby player, Steve was strong in many respects 'but I was physically weak,' he admits. 'I never did any upper-body work. I got stronger very quickly doing the programme. I started the chest press at 7.5-kilo dumbbells. By the end, I was pushing 25-kilo dumbbells. I had tripled my strength.'

He adds: 'Having been fortunate enough to play with and against some of the greatest rugby players around, such as Laurence Dallaglio and Martin Johnson, I was accustomed to working at the highest levels. I wanted to work with the best in my field.'

'PPP HEALTHCARE WERE PROVIDED WITH MEDICAL RECORDS OF PEOPLE WHO HAD BEEN COMPLETELY TRANSFORMED BY THE PROGRAMME.'

CASE STUDY #22
PETER ROACH

AGE 43 **OCCUPATION** MARKETING CONTROLLER
INCH LOSS AFTER SIX WEEKS
WAIST 2 **HIPS** 1 **CHEST** 1

Peter Roach was a marketing manager for PPP Healthcare when he recommended that the company sponsor Bodydoctor Fitness to create a proactive health-awareness programme. It was part of PPP's drive to position itself as a healthcare company and not just a private medical insurer.

Peter says, 'A colleague introduced me to Bodydoctor Fitness. He'd followed the programme at home from a manual and suggested that it might offer opportunities for the company. I have always had an interest in personal fitness. I checked out the website and ordered a manual. The ethos sat well with previous work that the company had conducted, promoting health awareness to primary school-aged children via an informative and fun curriculum-based resource called 'Alive & Active.' It was designed to help to overcome the 'couch potato' syndrome.

'I thought that Bodydoctor Fitness could help benefit existing customers, add value to new members and be promoted to the nation at large under a "Healthier Nation" banner. If the words in the Bodydoctor manual were true, then this programme could have a major impact.

'I arranged to meet David Marshall at his gym. I agreed to start training, under the watchful eye of David, to better understand how the programme worked and to experience it first-hand. I had lots of questions, and each time I was provided with an immediate, detailed answer, making me feel comfortable that this was a serious proposition.

'The immediate benefits of the programme were that I never felt tired after a session, I felt less stressed and had increased energy levels. The wider benefit was that the same programme I had undertaken could be completed by people from all walks of life. I started to get more into it, and wanted to determine if there was any clinical or user study that could prove some of the remarkable claims.

'I made a presentation to PPP with a proposal for a collaboration, with the aim of increasing the fitness of customers. There were many points that I liked. Safety was a key priority, the individual exercises were undertaken in a complementary process ("cleaning as you go") and it wasn't just about lifting heavy weights. And, finally, it worked. Just like Ronseal, it did what it said in the manual.'

Bodydoctor®

PART TWO

GETTING STARTED

NO MORE DELAY!
IT'S TIME TO:

LOSE 6 INCHES OFF YOUR WAIST
DOUBLE YOUR FITNESS
LOSE UP TO 1 STONE IN FAT
OVER THE NEXT SIX WEEKS.

Keep track!

Use a tape measure to measure yourself in the following places:

Shoulders: 2 in (5 cm) down from the tops of your shoulders

Chest: In line with the nipples

Waist: In line with the navel

Hips: Around the widest point of your bottom

Thigh: 2 in (5 cm) down from your crotch

Calf: Around the widest point

Arm: Halfway between your armpit and elbow

Weigh yourself and then PUT AWAY the scales. Do not use them for six weeks. After six weeks, re-measure in the same places.

THE TAPE MEASURE NEVER LIES. SCALES CAN.

Complete the data file

(see opposite)

NAME: _____

GENDER: _____ AGE: _____

WEIGHT: _____ HEIGHT: _____ BODY WEIGHT (if known): _____

DATA FILE

Please measure with a tape in the following places:

	START	6 WEEKS	12 WEEKS	18 WEEKS
SHOULDERS (2 inches down from the tops of your shoulders)				
CHEST (in line with nipples)				
WAIST (in line with belly button)				
HIPS (around the widest point of your bottom)				
THIGH (2 inches down from your crotch)				
CALF (around the widest point)				
ARM (halfway between your armpit and your elbow)				

	WEIGHT	REPS	WEIGHT	REPS	WEIGHT	REPS	WEIGHT	REPS
PEC DEC								
LAT PULL DOWN								
INCLINE DUMBELL PRESS								
STRAIGHT ARM PULLOVER								
SEATED SHOULDER PRESS								
SEATED LATERAL RAISE								
SEATED BICEP CURL								
TRICEP PRESS DOWN								
TRICEP BENCH DIP								
FULL PUSH UPS/ HALF PUSH UPS								
LUNGES								
SQUATS								

Cardiovascular work: Please keep a record of time and intensity of any of your cardiovascular work, i.e., machine, level of intensity, programme profile and duration.

NAME: _____

GENDER: _____ AGE: _____

WEIGHT: _____ HEIGHT: _____ BODY WEIGHT (if known): _____

DATA FILE

Please measure with a tape in the following places:

	START	6 WEEKS	12 WEEKS	18 WEEKS
SHOULDERS (2 inches down from the tops of your shoulders)				
CHEST (in line with nipples)				
WAIST (in line with belly button)				
HIPS (around the widest point of your bottom)				
THIGH (2 inches down from your crotch)				
CALF (around the widest point)				
ARM (halfway between your armpit and your elbow)				

	WEIGHT	REPS	WEIGHT	REPS	WEIGHT	REPS	WEIGHT	REPS
PEC DEC								
LAT PULL DOWN								
INCLINE DUMBELL PRESS								
STRAIGHT ARM PULLOVER								
SEATED SHOULDER PRESS								
SEATED LATERAL RAISE								
SEATED BICEP CURL								
TRICEP PRESS DOWN								
TRICEP BENCH DIP								
FULL PUSH UPS/ HALF PUSH UPS								
LUNGES								
SQUATS								

Cardiovascular work: Please keep a record of time and intensity of any of your cardiovascular work, i.e., machine, level of intensity, programme profile and duration.

THE BODYDOCTOR'S TOP 10 EXCUSES

1) I have over-exercised already this week.

2) I cannot be bothered.

3) It was a bit of a late night ...

4) I borrowed my boyfriend's open-top sports car last night and forgot to put the hood back up. Did you see the rain? I've gone into hiding.

5) My boyfriend says he's missing my curves.

6) My girlfriend doesn't like muscles.

7) The budgie has got out, and I can't leave the cat alone in the house.

8) What do you mean, my appointment was this morning?

9) I've just been to the hairdressers.

10) A tree uprooted itself and hit my car.

20 REASONS NOT TO MAKE EXCUSES

1) You will enjoy it when you start.

2) You will feel more energized.

3) You will look healthier.

4) People will comment on how well you look.

5) You will be able to wear that bikini.

6) You will not feel embarrassed by your holiday photographs.

7) People will stop asking when the baby is due.

8) You'll see your toes again.

9) You won't blush at the 'Excess Baggage' signs at airports.

10) Your life will change.

11) You will get a real kick when the weights you train with get heavier.

12) You really will be able to kick ass.

13) You will sleep better.

14) You'll be able to lift the tree off your bonnet.

15) You can wear those clothes at the back of the wardrobe.

16) You will stop feeling embarrassed in communal changing rooms.

17) Socializing will become more fun.

18) When a man approaches in a bar, you know he's coming over to you.

19) When someone sits on the bar stool beside you, it's not because it's the only one vacant.

20) You can fill the bath and not worry about the water overflowing when you get in.

THE GOLDEN RULES

Photocopy this page. Have it encapsulated. Take it with you to the gym. Have it by you when you work out at home. Make the Golden Rules your workout mantra. Repeat them to yourself. The Golden Rules keep you safe, and make you fit and healthy.

1. Work with weights that exhaust you between 20 and 25 repetitions. When you do this, you create a tremendous amount of heat in the muscle, which enables you to burn fat at source.

2. Breath is life. Breathe correctly and oxygenate your body. Breathe deeply with your lower stomach held in tight, as opposed to shallow lung breathing. Always exhale on the positive (exertion) movement: blow when you push a weight or when you pull a weight down on a cable. Inhale on the negative – on the way down or the release (suck). As you exhale, push the breath out of your stomach so you feel your stomach (abs) contract. Always work with your lower abs held in tight, not sucked in. If you train with your abs tight and pulled in, they will become tighter and firmer.

3. Keep hydrated. Drink a minimum of 1½ litres (eight glasses) of water a day. Always have a supply of water with you when you are training. Do not wait until you are thirsty to drink – by then you are probably already dehydrated. This workout is based on heat and breath, so you need to be hydrated at all times.

4. Exercise early in the day. When you exercise, you raise your metabolic rate (the number of calories you burn). If you exercise early in the day, your metabolism is raised for longer periods. When you sleep, your metabolism slows down. So when you work out early in the day, you burn more calories for longer, even after you have stopped training.

5. Eat before and after you exercise. You need to eat complex carbohydrates before you exercise, such as porridge oats, wholegrain bread or rye bread, and have protein within 1½–1¾ hours maximum after you've finished exercising (see the Nutrition section, page 195). It's also wise to have some snacks to hand in case you need to munch before or after your workout. Go for: dried apricots, trophy seed, nut and fruit bars and fruit – banana, apple, pear, cherries, berries, figs and dates. Buy medjoal (medjool) dates if you can – they contain high levels of glucose as well as fibre, which makes them excellent energy-boosters.

6. Work slowly. Work safely. If you try to run before you can walk, you fall over. Always start with a low weight and build up to 25 repetitions. When you can do 25 reps comfortably, increase the weight one increment.

Working speed with weights
2–3 seconds on the positive (push or pull) phase
4–6 seconds on the negative (return) phase.

How muscles get to work

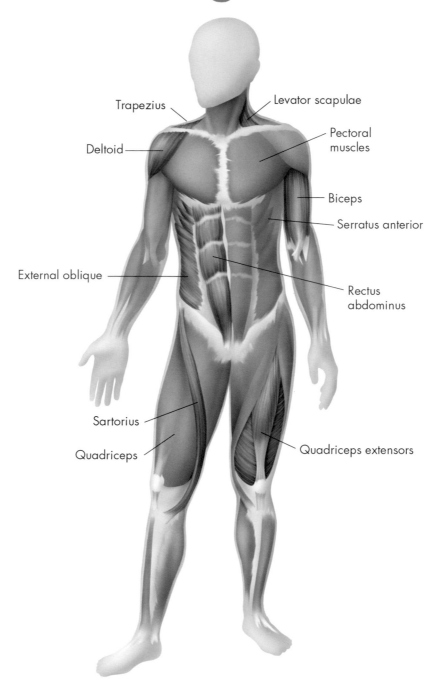

Trapezius

Levator scapulae

Deltoid

Pectoral
muscles

Biceps

Serratus anterior

External oblique

Rectus
abdominus

Sartorius

Quadriceps

Quadriceps extensors

Anterior view of the muscle-skeleton system

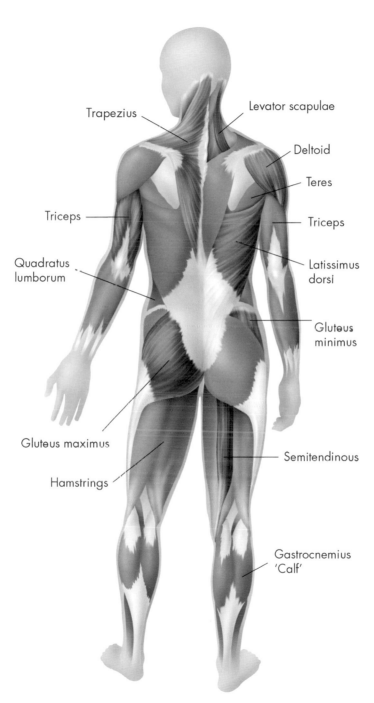

Trapezius

Levator scapulae

Deltoid

Teres

Triceps

Triceps

Quadratus
lumborum

Latissimus
dorsi

Gluteus
minimus

Gluteus maximus

Semitendinous

Hamstrings

Gastrocnemius
'Calf'

Posterior view of the muscle-skeleton system

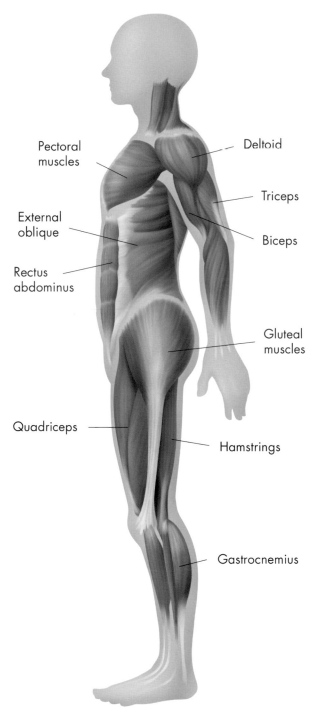

Pectoral
muscles

Deltoid

Triceps

External
oblique

Biceps

Rectus
abdominus

Gluteal
muscles

Quadriceps

Hamstrings

Gastrocnemius

Side view of the muscle-skeleton system

Now for the Science ...

For those science buffs among you, Sean Durkan, one of the osteopaths we refer clients to, sets out what the Bodydoctor Fitness Programme does for your body.

Each exercise has a positive and negative effect. The positive effect is the action –the contraction of specific muscles. When contraction is sustained for 25 repetitions, muscle is strengthened (the positive effect) and causes a negative effect, which is the shortening of muscle fibres and a build-up of toxins such as lactic acid and metabolites (the residual chemicals from cellular metabolism). These negatives have to be cleaned or removed, or we're left with shortened and sore muscles after a workout. The cleaning effect occurs in two ways: by thoroughly working all the muscle fibres, and by 'cleaning as you go' – when the next exercise acts to clean the muscles used in the previous exercise.

1 Cleaning the muscles
In all the exercises in the Bodydoctor exercise sequence, muscle is cleaned as it performs its full range of movement during the contraction and stretching phases of an individual exercise.

2 'Cleaning as you go'
The cleaning effect is enhanced when you perform the next exercise in the sequence, as this cleans up the negative effect – the contraction – by directly stretching the affected muscles from the previous exercise. The benefit is enhanced muscle function as strength and flexibility are increased in a balanced manner. This is 'cleaning as you go': the first nine exercises in the workout

sequence and the stretches work on this principle.

Reducing pain, improving circulation
The stretching cleans because it helps speed up the body's toxin transport system. Stretching releases residual muscle tension, which in turn eases the pressure on the blood vessels and lymphatic vessels. Their diameters increase, and toxins can flow more readily into the relevant lymphatic vessels and veins. The exercise sequence therefore promotes efficient detoxing as muscular pressure on the lymphatic drainage vessels is eased.

In the same way, stretching also helps improve the supply of nutrients and oxygen for muscle metabolism and reduces congestion in the veins. Blood pressure is defined by the heart rate multiplied by the body's resistance to blood flow – and the majority of this resistance is muscle tension. As stretching eases muscle tension, the heart doesn't have to work so hard, so you'll have more energy. Your body will also be in a more balanced state.

Stretching and cleaning the muscles also combats nerve irritation and resulting pain, as well as paresthesia, numbness and pins and needles. The build-up of toxins in the muscles being worked can activate the body's pain receptors, which inform the brain about the location of pain in the body: the tell-tale signs include muscle ache and soreness, which is often the 'morning after' result of a workout that isn't designed to work with your body. The Bodydoctor exercise regime is a muscular detox in itself so it's highly unlikely that you'll experience any residual pain, aches or stiffness after your workout, providing you follow it correctly and on a regular basis.

Protecting joints and bones

The exercise sequence also reduces the amount of abnormal wear and tear, degeneration of joints and inter-vertebral discs by improving muscular function and properly balancing the whole joint complexes involved. It also reduces abnormal leverage on joints, preventing subsequent straining or tearing of ligaments: for example, if certain muscles in a joint complex work harder or are stronger than the antagonistic muscle (the muscle that moves in the opposite direction), one side of the joint gets worn away faster than the other. Using the sequence balances the body, and improves your body's structure. This enhances your body's function as a whole, and helps you perform more efficiently.

Throughout the workout sequences, you'll see diagrams that show which muscles you're working during the exercise; it can be helpful to visualize your muscles as you do each movement, so you mentally focus on your technique. These diagrams are intended to be simple, so only the primary muscles involved are shown.

The story beneath the skin is, of course, more complex, as many principal muscles have more than one job. For example, parts of the same muscle in the shoulder girth have multiple actions due to the range of joints they connect with, such as the elbow, shoulder, rib cage and clavicle. So when we move any part of our arm, the majority of shoulder muscles contract; simply raising your arm activates 11 of the 17 major muscles in the shoulder girdle. For ease of reference therefore, only the primary muscles are illustrated to demonstrate the basic mechanics of each exercise.

What to wear

Don't be a fashion victim, or soon you may become a victim of injuries. Buy your trainers from respected sports shops. They are able to deal with people with problem feet. Some people walk on the outsides of their feet, whereas those with flat feet walk on the insides of their feet. Where trainers wear away indicates where the problems lie. They'll either wear evenly, or tend to wear on the outside or inside of the soles. A respected sports shop will tell you which trainers to buy accordingly.

The assistant should also be able to estimate the lifespan of a pair of trainers. For example, they'll know for how many miles your trainers will last. Old trainers can cause injuries due to lack of tread or a lack of support to the foot. Used regularly, good trainers will only be good for a limited time, so ask for recommendations of the better makes.

Remember to be astute; expensive trainers are a bit more expensive for a reason – as long as they're not a fashion con!

Your exercise clothes should be comfortable and loose fitting – and preferably cotton, so that the body can breathe. Nylon shorts are not only a style error but can cause chaffing between the legs.

And most importantly …

Keep drinking water throughout the whole programme. Keep a bottle beside you at all times (see the Golden Rules, page 73). And do not just drink when you feel thirsty – you'll probably be dehydrated by the time your body sends out this emergency signal. I recommend that you drink at least three-quarters of a pint of water (half a litre or so) for every half hour that you work out – and that is in ADDITION to the eight glasses you should be drinking as a matter of course.

Ready to start? Good …

CARDIOVASCULAR

WARMING UP

Now you probably have used these machines before and have finessed your technique, but indulge me for a few moments. I believe that the majority of people in gyms use them incorrectly and, as a consequence, do not get the maximum results. Try them my way! I promise you'll see a difference.

Bodydoctor®

Even top-class athletes warm up before they train. They don't just put on their shoes and go for a run. Rushing into training is a classic schoolboy error made by amateurs. But a short warm-up will increase body temperature, which allows the body fluids to flow better and, more importantly, lubricate the joints.

Start the Bodydoctor Fitness Programme with 10 minutes of moderate-intensity exercise. That means you should be working out at between 65 and 75 per cent of your maximum heart rate (see page 16). An ideal way to achieve this is by doing cardiovascular exercise, such as skipping; using a step machine, stationary bike or treadmill; or walking, jogging or cycling outdoors. Warming up means warming the body so you feel warm and a bit sweaty. You can't work muscle effectively in the absence of heat. But a warm-up is not intended to make the sweat pour off you so that you are too exhausted to carry on with the rest of the programme. Work at a steady, sustainable level – burning fat, even during the warm-up, is another key element to this programme.

Using the rowing machine

Place your feet into the stirrups and strap them in. Sit forward on your bottom (on the fleshy part) as opposed to the lower base of your spine (the coccyx). Take the handle in both hands. You are now in the starting position. Push away with both legs. Get used to the momentum of working with your legs for a few strokes. They will be doing most of the work for now, not your arms. When you have pushed yourself back, reach forward fully so that the bar reaches as near to your feet as possible. Then breathe out as you pull your hands (handle) into your gut (not your chest) pushing away with your legs. Breathe in as you pull yourself forward with your legs while reaching towards your feet with your hands. Get into a rhythm.

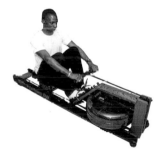 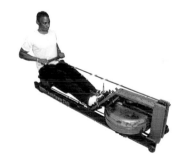

The idea is to let the motion of the rower and your legs and arms work in harmony. Keep your shoulders relaxed – you are not Noddy No-Neck.

DO NOT
Lean back as if you want to slam your shoulder blades into the floor behind you. You are not in the Oxford-Cambridge boat race; you don't have an 8-foot oar to pull through 20 feet of water!

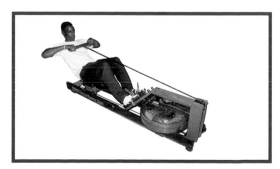

Using the treadmill

At Bodydoctor Fitness, we discourage running on the treadmill. It won't get you as good a result as walking at a fast pace on a gradient, and can also injure your body. When you run, you work the fast-twitch fibres in your muscles to give you leg speed and propel the joints forward. If you run on a treadmill, the fibres must act as secondary shock absorbers as each foot hits the belt. Walking lessens this impact and, in my opinion, when you walk on a gradient, you perform resistance exercise as you work to push your body weight up an incline. To match this resistance effect you would have to run up a gradient which is unsustainable for long periods.

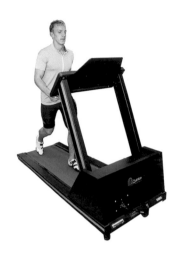

I won't patronize you by telling you how to walk. You should have learned that skill back in your first year. Just start by setting the speed to between 5 and 6 kilometres an hour. Take a long stride, keep the heel down as long as possible, then roll onto the ball of your foot. This movement uses the hamstring and buttocks. Now elevate the gradient from 5–10 per cent. Only go above 15 per cent if you are very fit! Keep your body towards the top of the slope. Keep walking, pushing off from the heels and then balls of your feet at all times.

DO NOT

Hold onto the rail in front of you! The treadmill is not a shopping trolley.

The Bodydoctor says: Work smarter, not harder!

Using the stepping machine

Place both feet on the pedals. Hold onto the stabilizing bars in front of you for balance only – and not as if you're hanging on for dear life. Keep your body upright at all times.

Lift your right foot to the top. As you place your weight onto the right foot, which makes it descend, lift up your left foot. Lift your right foot before it hits the floor and transfer your body weight to the left foot before it hits the top of the machine's range. You should aim to take deep steps.

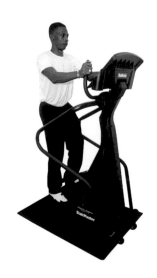

DO NOT

Hold onto the side rails and lean forward or stick out your bottom – you are not entering the Rear of the Year award! Do not flap your feet like a demented duck!

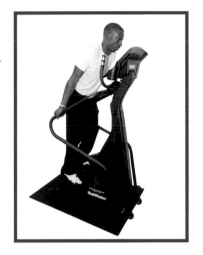

As you start working harder on a stepper, you will feel a natural inclination to copy all those so-called serious fitness fanatics around you. I mean, look at them. They're all bent forward.

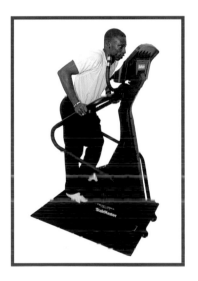

They're all huffing and puffing. They all look like sweaty beetroots, with their bums pushed out. All of them have the posture of a mobile battering ram and, hey, you're the only one who doesn't! Could you be right, and they be wrong? Well, you won't be going to see the back specialist in two weeks' time, but they might. They may appear to be working harder, but you are definitely working smarter Remember what the Bodydoctor says – it ain't what you do, it's how you do it.

Using the stationary bike

You have probably been riding a bicycle since you were five or six years old. And this one is much easier, because you don't have to maintain your balance at all times. Still, there are a few tips that I think are worth passing on.

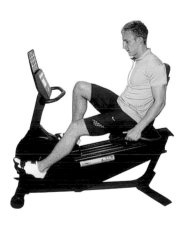

Ensure that your seat is positioned so your legs do not lock out as you cycle. Your leg should be slightly bent at the extended part of the movement. If the pedals are too far away, you will damage your knees. And finally, as the intensity increases and you start challenging yourself, resist the temptation to throw your head back! You're not in *Gone With the Wind*.

Outdoor warm-up

There will be some days when you fancy exercising outside in the open air, or you may want to do the programme from home but are not quite sure how to start. Jogging and power walking, although both beneficial, can be replaced with alternative ways of training outside (see page 175). However, for the purposes of warming up, 10–15 minutes of either activity at a heart rate of 60–75 per cent of your maximum will be the ideal way to warm up.

Your heart should be working at a comfortable pace, your body should be covered in a light sweat and you should be feeling warm. Then move on to a couple of light stretches (see below) to further loosen your body.

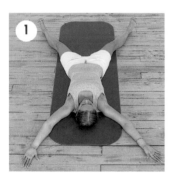

- I call this the 'X stretch'.
- Lay on your back, with your arms and legs extended out to the sides to make the shape of a big cross. Stretch your fingertips away from you, and stretch your legs downwards by pushing down from your heels. Stretch yourself out from all four points.
- Hold the stretch and breath normally.

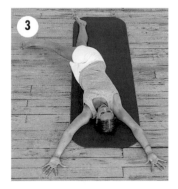

- Start by lying on the floor on your back in the 'X stretch'. Inhale deeply.
- As you exhale, keep your left arm straight and twist your body over to your right side so you get a twist at the waist. Keep both feet and your right arm anchored to the floor.
- Inhale as you stretch the fingertips of your left hand away from you, push down from your left and right heels, and stretch the fingertips of your right hand. Hold the position, breathing normally.
- Inhale as you relax and lay back on the floor.
- Repeat on the other side.

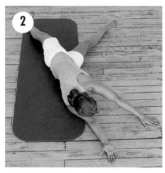

- Lie on your back in the 'X stretch' (see above) and inhale.
- Extend your right leg over your right thigh, and push your left heel down.
- Stretch both hands and feet away from your body. Hold the stretch and breathe normally.
- Inhale as you return to the cross position.
- Repeat with the left leg.

RESISTANCE TRAINING

This is probably the most important part of your programme.

Bodydoctor®

UPPER BODY GYM WORKOUT

Turn to page 110 if you are working out at home or if your gym does not have foot rests on its benches

On to the Serious Business

Three key points:

1 Breathing

You will have noticed that correct breathing is one of my Golden Rules (see page 73). When you exercise with weights, it is absolutely vital that you use the correct breathing technique. Here's my Golden Rule again: breathe deeply with your lower stomach held in tightly, as opposed to shallow lung breathing. Always breathe out when you are exerting yourself; that is when you push a weight or pull a weight down on a cable. As you exhale, push the breath out of your stomach so that you feel its muscles contract. Inhale as you return the weight to the starting position.

2 Carrying the weights from the rack to the bench

If there are no foot-rests on the benches in the gym, use the stability ball as in the home workout section. If there are no stability balls in your gym, workout at home or change your gym. This may sound like a silly point, but you can seriously injure yourself if you fail to transport weights correctly.

a) Incline position
Walk to the bench with a weight in each hand. Sit down with the weights resting on your thighs.

b) Recline position
Walk to the bench with a weight in each hand. Sit down with the weights resting on your thighs. As you lift one foot onto the footrest, recline while bringing the weights to rest on your chest, and then place the other foot on the footrest.

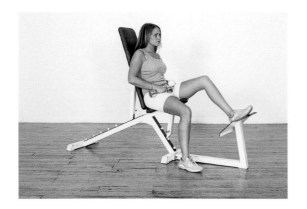 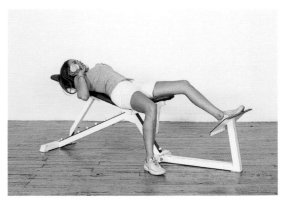

3 Sitting up on the bench after finishing the exercise

Again, it is important to do this correctly!

a) From the incline position
When you have finished the exercise, bring the weights down onto the tops of your thighs (where they meet your hips). Place both feet on the floor, then return the weights to the floor.

b) From the recline position
When you have finished the exercise, bring the weights down into the centre of your chest. Slide your hands down to your thighs. As you sit up, place one foot on the floor, then the other. With the weights still supported against your body, stand up.

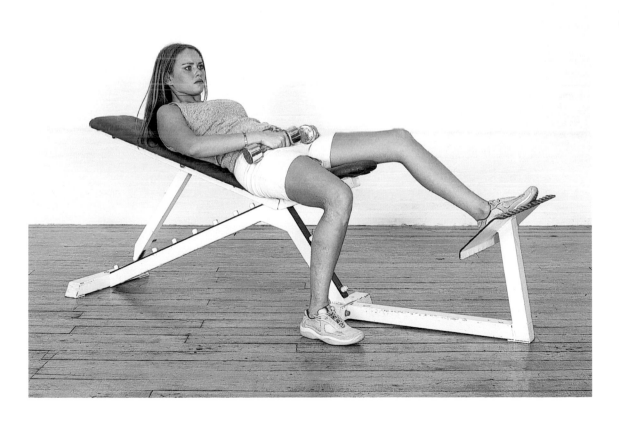

1

INCLINED CHEST FLIES

Strengthens the upper and inner chest muscles

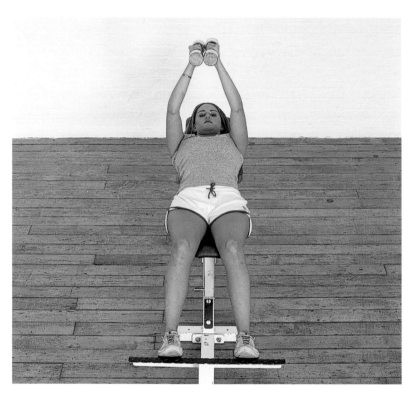

- Assume a lying position on the bench, with one dumbbell in each hand resting by your chest/armpit.
- Breathe out as you straighten both arms above your chest.

- Soften your elbows until your arms are bent at approximately 145 degrees, making a triangle above the centre of your chest.
- Maintain the shape throughout. Do not attempt to straighten your arms.

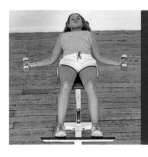

DON'T:
- Straighten your arms.
- Bring the weights down too fast.

WHAT AM I DOING?

Strengthening the pectoral muscles of the chest and the shoulder's anterior deltoid muscles on contraction. Stretching the muscles with the weight cleans them.

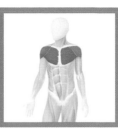

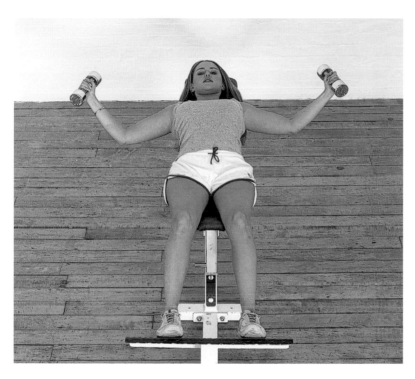

- Breathe in as you bring your arms and elbows to the side of your chest in an arc like movement – your elbows should be parallel to your back.
- Breathe out as you return the weights above your head.

- When you have reached 25 repetitions (or fatigue), bring the weights back down to the side of your chest/armpit, and let them slide back down to your thigh/hip as you return safely to an upright position (see page 87).

- Allow your arms to come down too far – you do not want to feel your shoulders squeezing.

LAT PULL-DOWN

Strengthens the side of the back, shoulders and arms

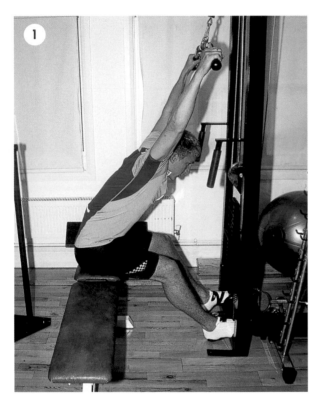

- With the bench level take a wide grip on the lat pull-down bar.
- Sit back on your bench and lean forward from your waist, not your back.
- Keep your spine straight.

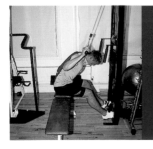

DON'T:
- Sit upright with your back rounded and your head craning forward.
- Allow the bar to move up very fast.

The primary function is to strengthen the latissimus dorsi, the inferior fibres of the trapezius and rhomboids. The secondary action is to clean and stretch the pectoral and deltoid muscles from the previous exercise.

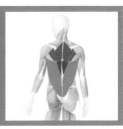

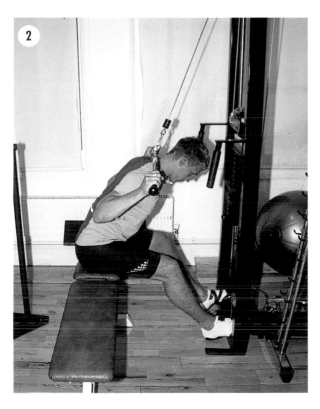

- Breathe out as you pull the bar down behind your head.
- Keep your body leaning forward, so that your chest is going towards your thighs.
- Do not have a bend in your back.

- When you have reached 25 repetitions (or fatigue), hold the bar against the back of your neck and squeeze for 10 seconds.
- Release slowly.

- **Propel yourself forward from the shoulders to bring the bar down.**

3

INCLINED DUMBBELL PRESS

Strengthens the upper chest, front of shoulders, backs of the arms and the gut

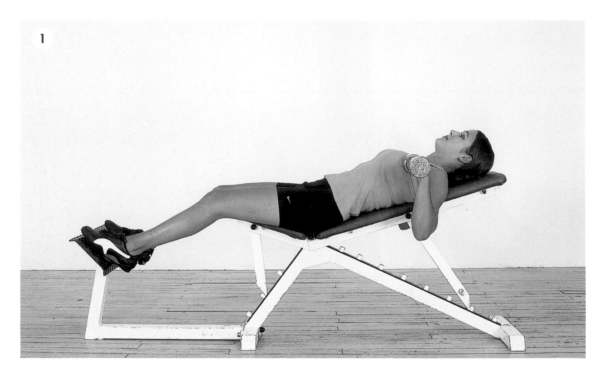

1

- Assume a lying position on the bench, with one dumbbell in each hand resting by your chest/armpit.
- Position the bench so the seat and back support are slightly raised, on the first notch up from level.

From the side, the bench should look like the hands of a clock reading ten to two.
- Lie back with a dumbbell in each hand at chest height.

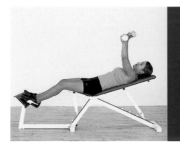

DON'T:
- Push your hands out round in a circular motion.
- Allow the weights to come down by picking up speed.

WHAT AM I DOING?

Strengthening the pectoral muscles in your chest, the deltoid muscles of the shoulder and triceps, located at the back of the upper arm. The secondary benefit is that you stretch and clean out the back and shoulder muscles from the previous exercises.

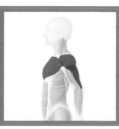

2

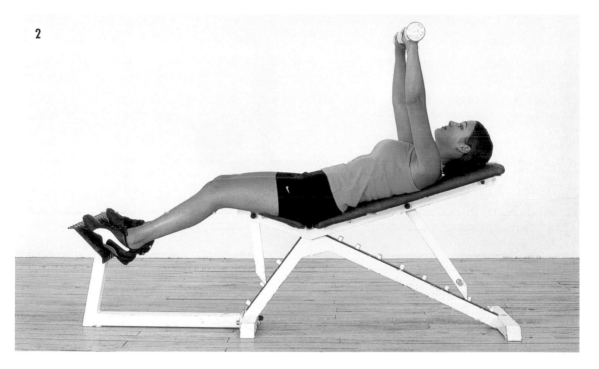

- With your palms facing forward and wrists firm, breathe out as you extend your arms above your chest.
- Imagine that you are making a triangle with two wide points at the bottom, going into a peak at the top.
- Breathe in as you pull back from the peak to return to the original base-of-triangle position.
- When you have reached 25 repetitions (or fatigue), bring the weights back down to the side of your chest/armpit, and let them slide back down to your thigh/hip as you return safely to an upright position (see page 87).

- Allow either of your knees to turn outwards or inwards.
- Push the weights above your chin or your stomach.

4

STRAIGHT-ARM PULL-OVER

A counterbalancing exercise to stretch and relax all the muscles in the upper body

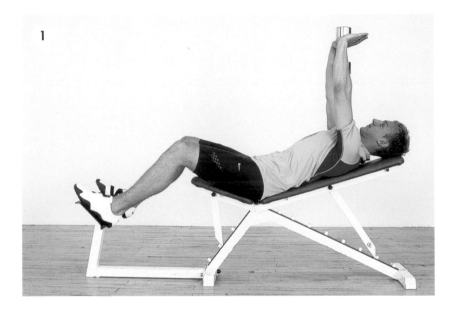

- Stay in the same position as required for the Inclined Dumbbell Press (see page 92).
- Cradle a weight between both hands, with your palms flat and facing upwards.

- Extend the arms above your chest until they are almost locked, yet still slightly soft.
- Bend your wrists back until they are almost parallel with the floor. Maintain the elbow position.

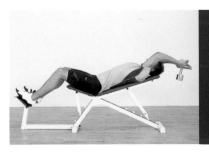

DON'T:
- Let your arms buckle at the elbows.
- Bend backwards from the elbow when the weight is extended beyond the head.

WHAT AM I DOING?

Strengthening the pectoral muscles of the chest, the teres major and latissimus dorsi muscles of the back and the serratus muscles of the ribcage in a different plane of direction from the previous exercises. The secondary benefit is that you stretch and clean out the pectoral, deltoid and tricep muscles from the previous exercises.

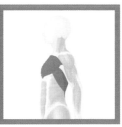

2

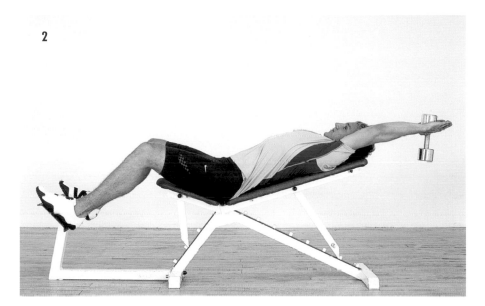

- Breathe in as you arc the weight behind your head until your forearms and upper arms are level and in line with your upper body.
- Ensure that your wrists straighten out so that your forearms and upper arms maintain the alignment with your upper body. Your wrist should be acting as a hinge.
- Maintain a straight line parallel with the floor and feel a stretch in your chest, back, shoulders and underarms.

- If your flexibility does not allow you to go this far, stop when you have reached a comfortable stretch.
- Breathe out as you return the weight to its starting position.
- When you have reached 25 repetitions (or fatigue), bring the weight back down to the side of your chest/armpit, and let it slide back down to your thigh/hip as you return safely to an upright position (see page 87).

Upper body gym workout

5

SEATED SHOULDER PRESS

Strengthens the shoulders and backs of the arms

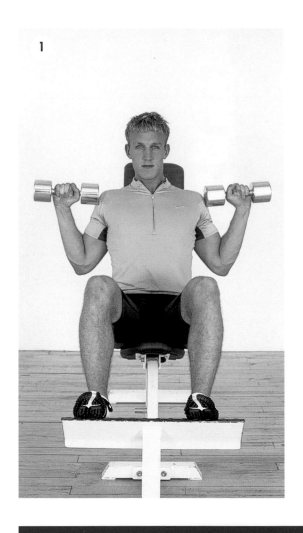

1

- Position the seat of the bench slightly up and the back of the chair almost straight up. From the side, the bench should look like the hands of a clock set at five to two.
- Sit with your feet positioned apart. Imagine that you are making a triangle as you conduct this exercise.
- Hold a weight in each hand at shoulder height.

DON'T:

- Allow the weights to move in front or behind your head.
- Allow the weights to come down by picking up speed.
- Cut down the range of your movement.
- Push your hands out and round in a circular motion.

WHAT AM I DOING?

Strengthening the deltoid muscles of the shoulder and the trapezius muscles on the upper shoulder towards the back of the neck. The secondary benefit is that you stretch and clean the pectorals, teres major, latissimus and serratus muscles from the previous exercises.

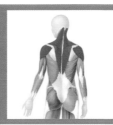

2

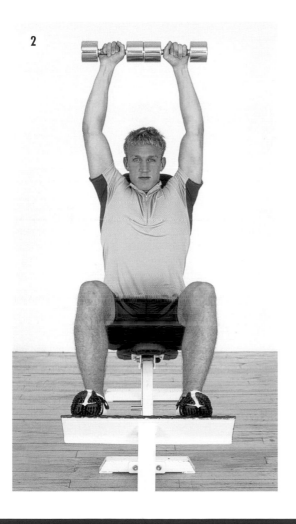

- Breathe out as you push the weights above your head so that they touch together above the crown. Resist the temptation to look up.
- Breathe in as you bring the weights down to touch your shoulders at the bottom.
- When you have reached 25 repetitions (or fatigue), bring the weights back down to the side of your chest/armpit, and let them slide back down to your thigh/hip (see page 87).

6

SEATED LATERAL RISE

Strengthens the shoulders, upper back and backs of the arms

1

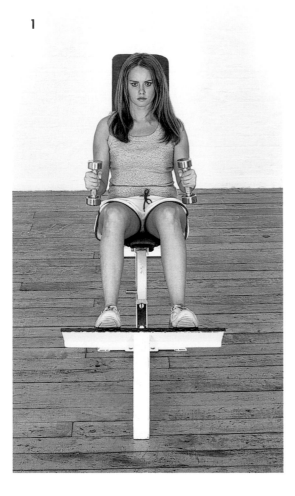

- You can visualize this exercise. Imagine that you are not holding any weights, and then let your arms float up until they are parallel with your shoulders. Now imagine the movement with your arms locked at right angles. It's as simple as that.
- Keep the seat in the same position as for the Seated Shoulder Press (see page 96).
- Bend your arms and bring the weights up until your arms form a right angle.

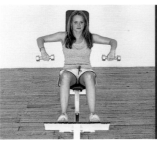

DON'T:
- Try and jerk the weights up like a chicken.
- Allow the weights to come down by picking up speed.

WHAT AM I DOING?

Strengthening the deltoid muscles of the shoulder. The secondary benefit is that you clean and stretch the pectoral muscles, latissimus muscles and triceps from the previous exercises.

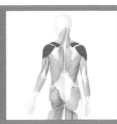

2

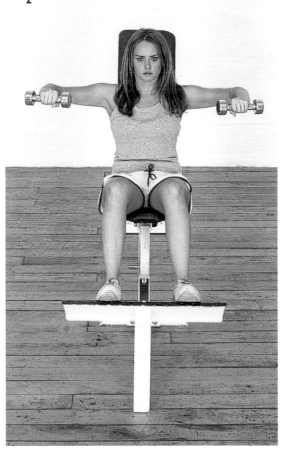

- Breathe out as you raise the weights up until your hands, forearms, upper arms and elbows are all level with your shoulders, yet still locked at right angles. This should be a smooth, sweeping movement. There should be no independent movement of the wrist, forearm, upper arm or head.
- Check the weights – they should be horizontal, parallel with each other.
- Breathe out as you return to the starting position.
- Now check the weights: both should be vertical.
- When you are about to reach 25 repetitions (or fatigue), hold the weights in position for a few seconds on your final upward sweep. Bring your arms down to the sides. Lean forward from the waist, arms hanging forward. Let head and neck relax. Allow your muscles to spread and stretch. Breathe in and out.

- **Cut down on the range of movement.**
- **Allow your knees to turn outwards or inwards.**

7

SEATED BICEP CURL

Strengthens the arms

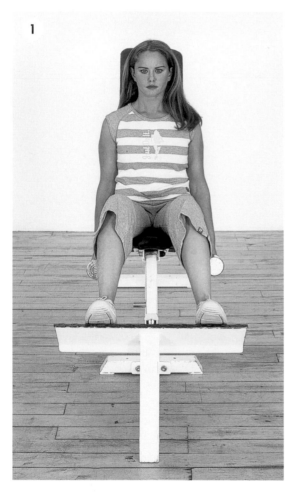

1

- Retain the same seated position as for the Seated Lateral Raise (see page 98).
- Tuck in your stomach.
- Soften your neck.
- Hold the weights down by your side, with palms facing inwards.
- Remember that your arm is a hinge; you should only work the elbow and below. The upper arm should remain tucked into the side at all times during this exercise.

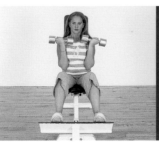

DON'T:

- Cut down the range of movement.
- Allow the weights to come down by picking up speed.

Bodydoctor

WHAT AM I DOING?

Strengthening the elbow flexors – the biceps. The secondary benefit is to stretch out the deltoids and tricep muscles from the previous exercises.

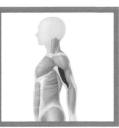

2

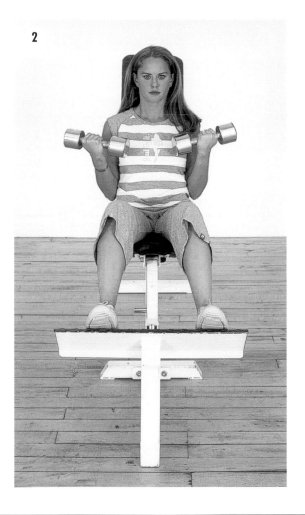

- Breathe out as you curl the weights towards your shoulders. The palms should face the shoulders at the end of the movement.
- Breathe in as you lower the arms until they are fully extended, and uncurl the weights.
- When you have reached 25 repetitions (or fatigue), bring the weights back down to your sides (see page 87).

- Allow either of your knees to turn inwards or outwards.
- Allow your arms to swing behind you when they come down.

- Swing your arms on the way up.
- Thrust your arms into position.

8

TRICEP PRESS-DOWN

Strengthens the backs of the arms and the shoulders

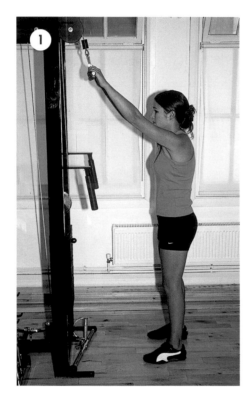

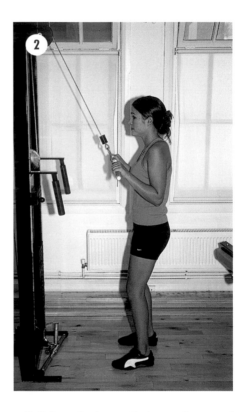

- Grasp the bar in your hands, with your thumbs on top.
- Position yourself so that your arms are fully extended from your body when you are holding the bar.
- Your feet should be about a hip-width apart, with one foot slightly in front of the other.

- Pull down the bar so that your elbows and upper arms tuck into your sides.
- Tuck in your stomach and soften your knees.
- Keep your chin up.

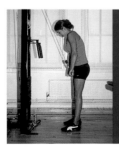

DON'T:
- Allow your upper arms to move forward.
- Allow your elbows to come out or away from your sides.

WHAT AM I DOING?

Strengthening the triceps, on the back of the upper arms. The secondary benefit is that you stretch the biceps from the previous exercises.

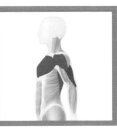

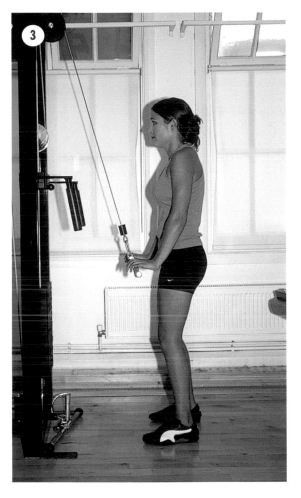

- Breathe out as you push the bar down until your arms are fully extended. As you push down, loosen your grip so that your hands are outstretched with your palms resting on the bar.
- Breathe in as you slowly return the bar to position 2 at chest height.
- Return your hands to a loose-grip position, keeping the thumb on top at all times.
- Do 25 repetitions (or until fatigued).

- Allow the bar to come up too fast.
- Round your shoulders and push down using your body weight.

- Allow your stomach to take more than minimal strain.

9

TRICEP BENCH DIP

Strengthens the backs of the arms and the shoulders

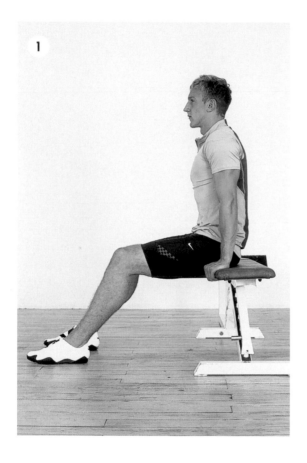

- Alter the bench setting so that it is completely flat.
- Sit on it with your hands grasping the edges by the sides of your thighs. Your wrists should be facing behind you. They should not be at an angle.
- Shift your buttocks until you are sitting just off the edge of the bench with your knees bent at 90 degrees. Your feet should be flat on the floor.

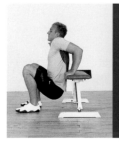

DON'T:

- Move your bottom and back more than an inch from the edge of the bench.
- Sit your weight down — you should lower it.

WHAT AM I DOING?

Strengthening the triceps (at the back of the upper arm), the pectoralis major muscles of the chest and the deltoids, of the shoulder. The secondary benefit is that you stretch and clean the pectorals and latissimus dorsi from the previous exercises.

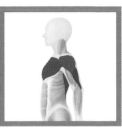

2

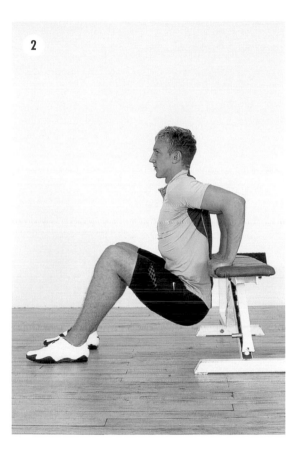

- Lower yourself off the bench by bending your elbows until the edge of the bench is level with your mid to lower back. Use only your arms to achieve this.
- Push yourself back up by straightening your arms.
- Repeat the movement.
- Do 25 repetitions (or until fatigued) without sitting back on the bench.

- Push up from the hips, thighs or legs.
- Let your shoulder and ears touch each other.

10
HALF PRESS-UP
Strengthens the chest, arms and shoulders

1

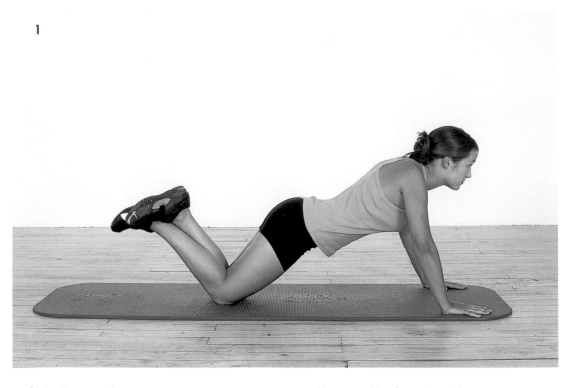

- Sit back on your knees.
- Walk your hands forward until your body is on all fours.
- Move your knees slightly apart and lock your feet.

- Move your hips forward and down.
- Your head, back and both legs should be in a straight line.

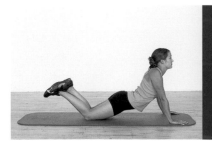

DON'T:
- Push up from your bottom.
- Arch your back.

WHAT AM I DOING?

Strengthening the pectoral muscles, deltoids and a whole host of muscles, including the abdominal muscles and gluteal muscles of the hips and buttocks.

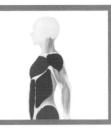

2

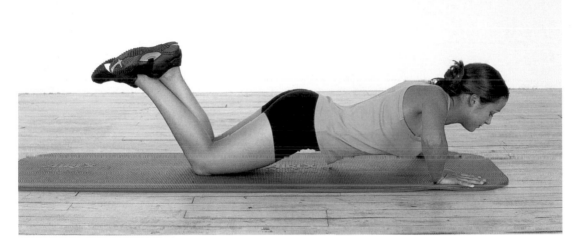

- Take your hands out slightly wider.
- Breathe in as you dip down.
- Breathe out as you go up.

- There should be no independent movement of the torso. The movement is generated by your arms.
- Do 25 repetitions (or until fatigued).

• Let your stomach sag — remember, tight abs!

FULL PRESS-UP

Strengthens the chest, shoulders, arms, back, stomach and thighs

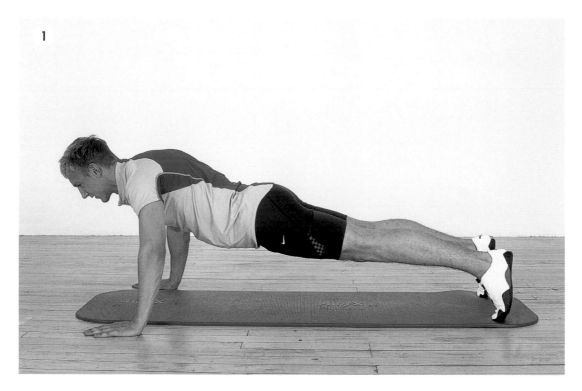

1

- Start from the basic half press-up position, with your knees on the floor and your upper body in a straight line.
- Move your hands further forward, until they are in line with your shoulders.

- Lift your knees off the floor.
- Balance your weight on your toes.
- Keep your head, neck, back, bottom and legs in a straight line.

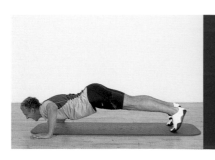

DON'T:
- Push up from your bottom.
- Let your stomach sag – remember, tight abs!

WHAT AM I DOING?

Strengthening the pectoral muscles, deltoids and a range of other muscles including the abdominal muscles and gluteal muscles of the buttocks and hips.

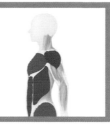

2

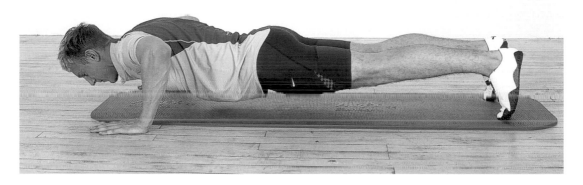

- Breathe out as you push your body up.
- Breathe in as you lower yourself to just above the floor. The movement is achieved by bending your arms at the elbows.
- Do 25 repetitions (or until fatigued). When 25 repetitions becomes easy, pause for one minute then do a repeat set.

- **Arch your back.**
- **Allow your knees to touch the floor.**

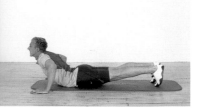

Now move on to the lower body workout on page 140.

Bodydoctor®

RESISTANCE TRAINING

You'll need a Swiss ball (stability ball) for your home workout. Always use a high-quality anti-burst ball for safety (if punctured, it deflates slowly). Clear away anything in the room you would not want to fall towards.

Exercising correctly on a Swiss ball is an art in itself and one that should not be taken lightly. I strongly suggest that you attempt challenges one and two before you attempt the resistance exercises on the ball. When you feel comfortable with your stability and balance, go through all the exercises using imaginary dumbbells. You may be very experienced at exercise and be familiar with resistance training, but that's not a worthy preparation for stability work. Be complacent with the ball at your peril.

UPPER BODY HOME WORKOUT

The correct seated position for the Swiss ball

Stand in front of the Swiss ball, with your feet positioned a hip-width apart. With your head upright, lower yourself until you are sitting on the Swiss ball. Your feet, which should be facing forward, should still be positioned a hip-width apart. Walk yourself forward off the ball until you feel that you are about to fall off — and then walk back 2 in (5 cm). Correct your feet so that they are a hip-width apart. Your heels should be directly below your knees. As you look down, your knees should also be a hip-width apart. Now let's check out the rest of the body. Make sure that your stomach and belly button are tightly sucked in so that you have a slight tension in your midriff. Correct your spine. Do not arch — imagine that you have a thread drawing you up towards the ceiling. Check your feet again (they tend to wander off on their own!). Keep your chin up and look forward. You are now sitting in the perfect position in which to perform exercises 5, 6 and 7 — the shoulder press, lateral raise and bicep curl (see pages 126, 128, 130).

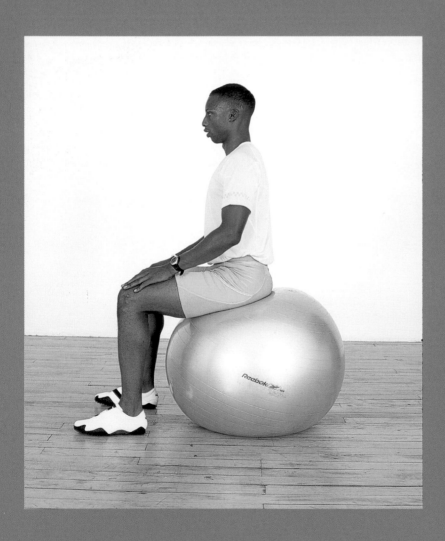

The correct recline (bridge) position for the Swiss ball

Stand with your back to the ball, with your feet a hip-width apart. Now sit on the ball with your head upright and your back straight. Walk slowly forwards until your lower back, then middle back and shoulder blades make contact with the ball. From this position, bring your feet slightly back so that your heels are directly below your knees. Keep your knees and feet a hip-width apart. Move forward slightly so that your head and neck make contact with the ball. Then raise your pelvis and hips, clench your buttocks and tighten your stomach. This is the bridge position.

1) Check again that your heels are directly beneath your knees. In this position, imagine that you have weights in your hands and perform the movements as described with dumbbells, but without dumbbells, until you feel comfortable and not tired. When you can perform each movement 25 times with no weights, just an imaginary dumbbell, you are ready to progress to working with dumbbells. It is vital that you can maintain the position and achieve core stability without feeling too much fatigue. The areas that tend to tire out first are your buttocks and lower back. If this happens, lower your buttocks towards the floor as you lift your head.

2) When your lower back is in contact with the ball, put the weights down and walk yourself backwards until you are back up on the ball in a seated position. Do this as soon as you feel fatigued — don't risk injuring your body. As you practice, you'll find that you can go longer without the need to sit back on the ball.

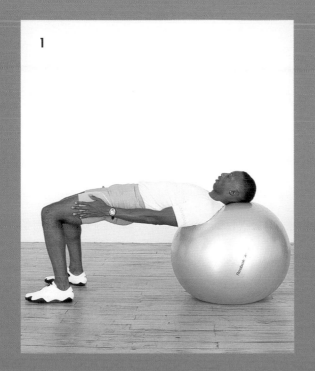

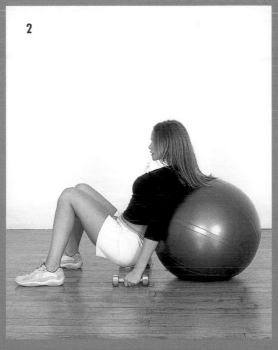

1: CORE STABILITY

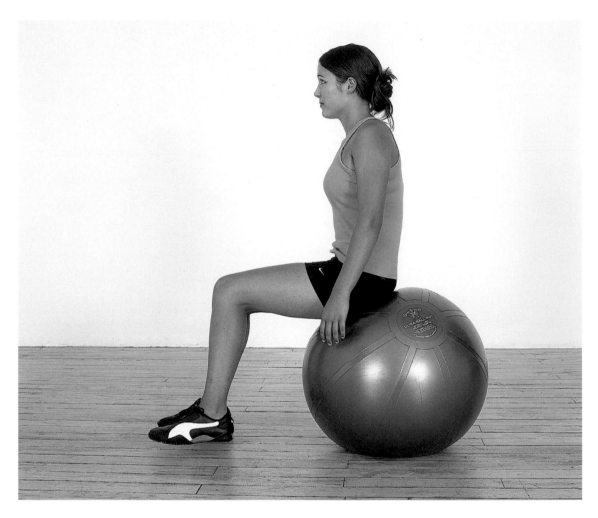

- Take up the correct seated position (see page 112). Let your hands hang loosely by the side of the ball; they should not grip it. Keep your shoulders relaxed and your head held high. You should feel a slight tension in your stomach.
- Attempt to slowly raise either your right or left foot approximately an inch from the ground. Make sure that your back keeps its natural shape and does

not hollow, and that you don't release the tension from your stomach.
- The idea is not to wobble or allow your weight to shift from right to left.
- Simply try to lift one foot off the ground while maintaining the correct posture. You should feel a slight tension in your stomach and your thighs will begin to burn. This is core stability at work.

2: THE CRUNCH

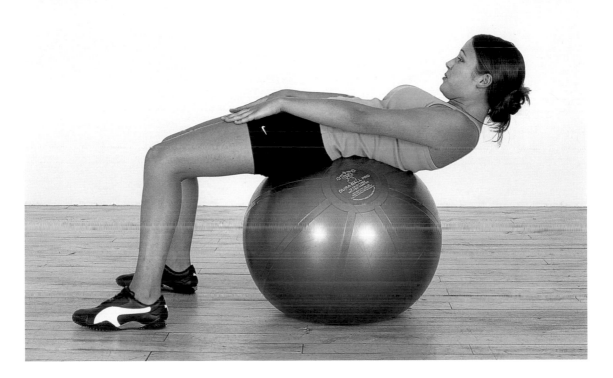

- From the seated position, walk yourself forward so that your lower spine is supported.
- Hold the tension in your stomach.
- Place your palms on your thighs. Now slide yourself forward so that you use your abs to curl, touching the tips of your fingers to your knees.
- Allow yourself to roll back gently so that the middle of your spine is supported by the ball, and your hands rest on the middle of your thighs.

- Slide forward again to touch your knees.
- This is a crunch on the Swiss ball.
- Your feet should be slightly forward of your knees, rocking forwards and backwards from the middle of your thighs to the ends of your knees.

3: BALANCE ON ALL FOURS

1

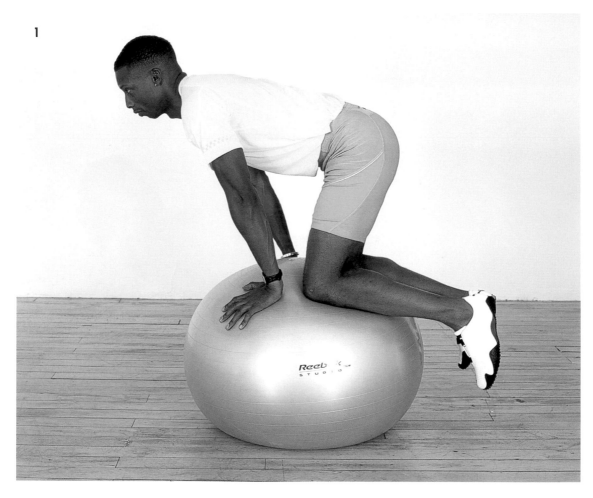

- Do not attempt this unless you have excellent balance and fast reflexes, because you may fail to get into position and fall off the ball. The exercise may not appear challenging on paper, but balancing on the Swiss ball demands complete core stability.
- Stand slightly in front of the ball, then attempt to slowly balance on it on all fours.

- Position your left hand then right hand, followed by your left and right knee until you are on all fours on the ball. Keep your stomach tensioned and do not allow your back to round upwards. You control the sway of the ball by moving your hips, knees and hands to maintain balance. The objective is not to hit the floor. Be safe and sensible!

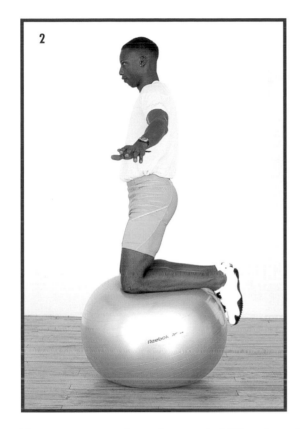

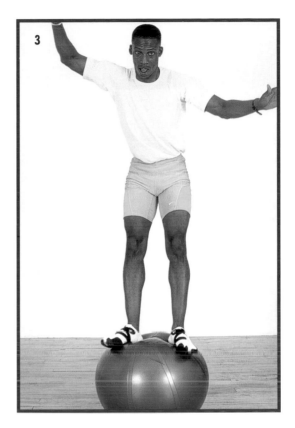

These are examples of core stability at work and are not to be attempted.

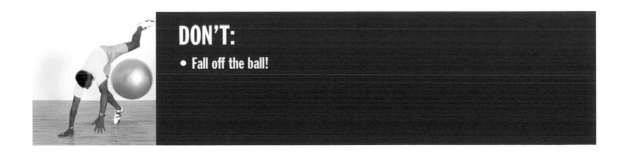

DON'T:

• Fall off the ball!

CHEST FLIES

Strengthens the upper and inner chest muscles

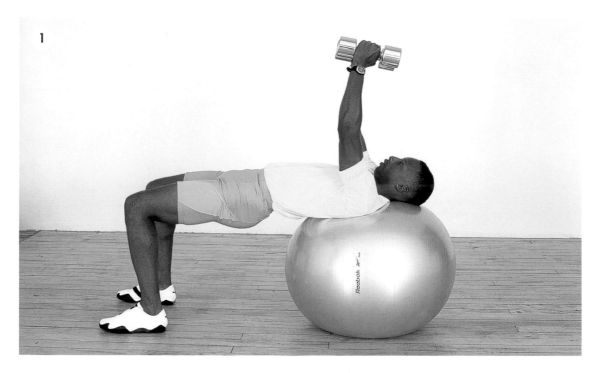

1

- Get into the Bridge position on the Swiss ball: with your feet positioned a hip-width apart, lower yourself with head upright until you are sitting on the ball. Make sure your feet are still a hip-width apart and you are looking forward. Now slowly walk forward, lowering yourself onto the ball until your shoulder blades touch the ball. Pause for a second. From there, walk very slowly forward until your neck and head are both finally supported by the ball. Bring your heels back directly under your knees, making sure they are also hip-width apart.

- Create tension in your stomach and raise your hips so they are level with your shoulders and knees, making sure your head stays comfortably on the ball. Shoulder blades, head and neck should all be supported by the ball. Your feet should be directly below your knees and your knees should be hip-width apart, in alignment with your feet.

- Check again that you have correct tension in your stomach and that your hips have not dipped. You've achieved the Bridge position. From here, bring the dumbbells to your chest. You are now ready to perform the chest flies.

- Straighten your arms above your chest, so that your palms and wrists are facing each other. Soften your elbows until your arms are bent at approximately 145 degrees, making a triangle above your chest. Maintain the shape of your arms throughout. Do not attempt to straighten or close your arms.

Strengthening the pectoral muscles of the chest and the shoulder's anterior deltoid muscles on contraction. Stretching the muscles with the weight cleans them.

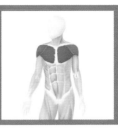

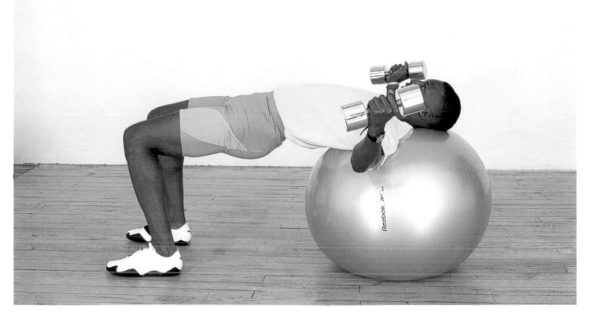

2

- Breathe in as you bring your arms and elbows down to the sides of your chest in an arc, so that the backs of your arms just touch the sides of the Swiss ball.
- Breathe out as you push back up to the start position.
- Breathe in as you bring your arms down to touch the sides of the ball. Breathe out as you return to the position above the centre of your chest.

- Do 25 repetitions (or until fatigued), then bring the weights down to the centre of your chest, move your hands down to your hips and lower your hips until your lower back makes contact with the ball.
- From this position, put the weights down on the floor, walk back onto the ball until you are in the seated position, and stand up.

2

LAT PULL-DOWN

Strengthens the side of the back, shoulders and arms

1

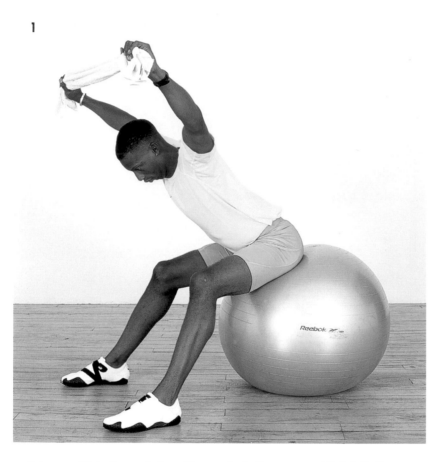

- Get yourself into the seated position on the ball (see page 112). With a towel gripped firmly in both hands above your head, pull it taut until it is about 1½–2 ft (half a metre or so) wide. This is your starting position.

WHAT AM I DOING?

Strengthening the latissimus dorsi and rhomboid muscles of the back, and the inferior fibres of the trapezius (located on the upper shoulder and towards the back of the neck). The secondary benefit is that you clean and stretch the pectoral and deltoid muscles from the previous exercise.

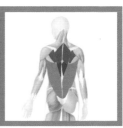

2

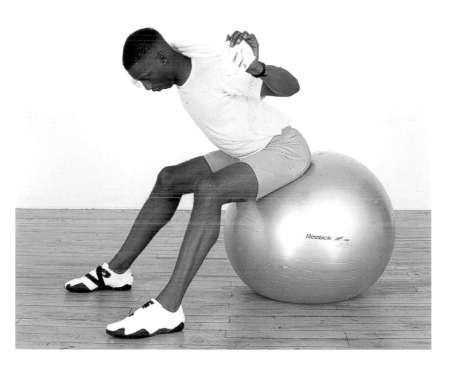

- Lean forward from the waist and, keeping the tension in the towel, breathe out as you pull it down behind your head so that it touches the back of your neck.

- Breathe in as you extend your arms back.
- Keep the towel taut at all times.
- Do 25 repetitions (or until fatigued).

3

CHEST DUMBBELL PRESS

Strengthens the upper chest, front of shoulders, backs of arms and the gut

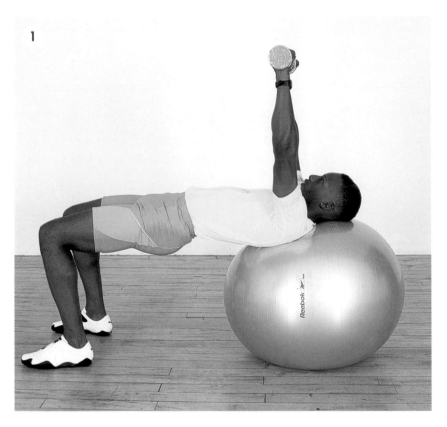

1

- Take two dumbbells – remember to start with light weights!
- Place on your thighs, adjacent to your stomach, as you sit in the starting position.
- Walk forwards very slowly until your shoulder blades and neck rest on the ball. This is the Bridge position (see page 113).
- Raise the weights up above the centre of your chest.
- Soften your elbows and make sure that the inside edge of both wrists face each other.

WHAT AM I DOING?

Strengthening the pectoral muscles in your chest, the deltoid muscles of the shoulder and triceps, located at the back of the upper arm. The secondary benefit is that you stretch and clean out the back and shoulder muscles from the previous exercises.

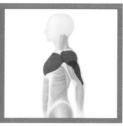

2

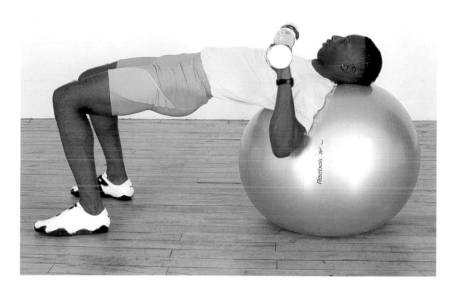

- Breathe in as you bring your arms out, maintaining the angle until the backs of your arms make contact with the Swiss ball.
- Breathe out as you return your arms to the starting position.
- Your elbows should be soft when they are above your chest.
- Make sure at all times that you do not lower hips. Maintain the integrity of your position. (Any exercise on a ball requires that you maintain a stable position – see the core stability exercise on page 113.) As soon as your stability starts to wander, it's

time to stop exercising or move to a lighter weight.
- Do 25 repetitions (or until fatigued). On the final repetition, bring the weights down into your chest.
- Lower your hips until your buttocks make contact with the front of the ball, and simultaneously raise your head.
- Put the weights down on the floor, then slowly walk back up into a seated position.
- Rest before embarking upon the next exercise. Rest means letting your stomach, lower back, buttocks and thighs recover.

Upper body home workout

123

4

STRAIGHT-ARM PULL-OVER

A counterbalancing exercise to stretch and relax all muscles in the upper body

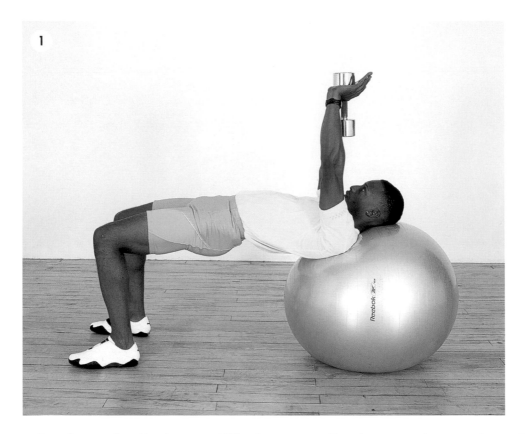

- From the seated position (see page 112), take one dumbbell and hold it against your stomach.
- Walk to the recline position (see page 113).
- Cradle the dumbbell in the palms of your hands.

- Extend your arms above your chest until they are almost locked, but still soft.
- Your wrists should be bent back so that the dumbbell is parallel to floor, but pointing to ceiling.

WHAT AM I DOING?

Strengthening the pectoral muscles of the chest, the teres major and latissimus dorsi muscles of the back and the serratus muscles of the ribcage in a different plane of direction from the previous exercises. The secondary benefit is that you stretch and clean out the pectoral, deltoid and tricep muscles from the previous exercises.

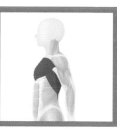

2

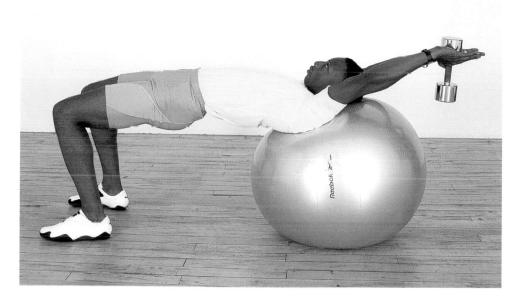

- Breathe in as you bring the dumbbell down in an arc behind your head until you feel a comfortable stretch in your armpits, inner arms and triceps, and the backs of your shoulders make contact with the ball.
- Hold for one second.
- Make sure that your wrists don't flop backwards.
- Breathe out as you bring your arms back to the starting position.

- When you feel yourself getting tired in a mid-section, place the dumbbell on the middle of your chest. Lower your hips until the back of your buttocks touch the front of the ball as you simultaneously lift the weight off your body and place the dumbbells on floor.
- Do 25 repetitions (or until fatigued).

5

SEATED SHOULDER PRESS

Strengthens the shoulders and the backs of the arms

1

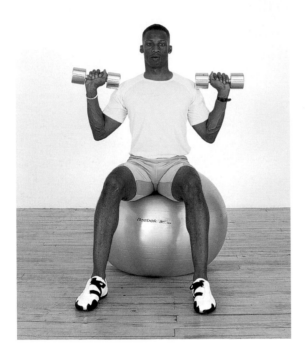

- Take the dumbbells and sit correctly on the ball (see page 112).
- Your heels should be under your knees.
- Move the dumbbells to either side of the ball.
- Your palms should be facing in towards the ball.
- Raise the dumbbells to either side of your shoulders. They should not be resting on your chest or behind your head.
- Make sure that your elbows are in a deep position.
- Keep your stomach tense and your head forward.
- Check your feet! Remember, they have a mind of their own.
- The dumbbells should not be in front of your head or behind. They should come up directly past your ears.

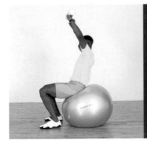

DON'T:
- Allow the weights to move in front or behind your head.
- Cut down the range of your movement.

WHAT AM I DOING?

Strengthening the deltoid muscles of the shoulder and trapezius muscles on the upper shoulder towards the back of the neck. The secondary benefit is that you stretch and clean the pectorals, teres major, latissimus dorsi and serratus muscles from the previous exercises.

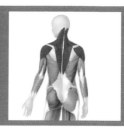

2

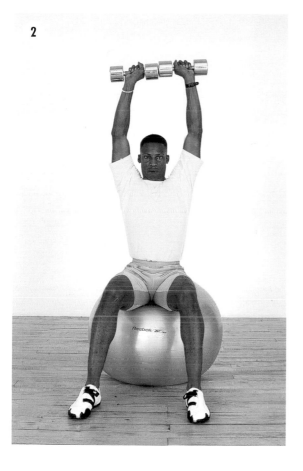

- Breathe out as you push the dumbbells into a triangular position, closing directly above your head.
- Breathe in as you follow the triangle position down until the dumbbells again reach your shoulders.
- Check your position has not altered and your back is not arched.
- Do 25 repetitions (or until fatigued).
- If you feel any stress in your back or stomach it means that you're not in the correct position, so stop the exercise. Lower the weights to your hips. Walk back onto the ball and, when you are seated comfortably, stand up.

- Push your hands out and round in a circular motion.
- Let your heels come too close to the ball.

- Allow the weights to come down by picking up speed.
- Allow either of your knees to turn outwards or inwards.

6

SEATED LATERAL RAISE

Strengthens the shoulders, upper back and backs of the arms

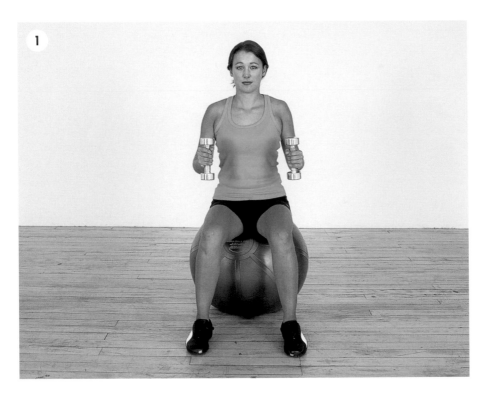

- Sit on the ball in the correct position (see page 112) with a dumbbell in each hand.
- Sit with the weights hanging by the side of your thighs.

- Bend your arms, and bring up the weights until your arms form a right angle.

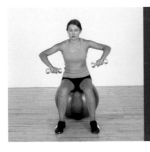

DON'T:
- Try and jerk the weights up like a chicken.
- Cut down on the range of movement.

WHAT AM I DOING?

Strengthening the deltoid muscles of the shoulder and the supraspinatus muscles around the shoulder blade. The secondary benefit is that you clean and stretch the pectoral muscles, latissimus dorsi muscles and triceps from the previous exercises.

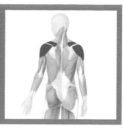

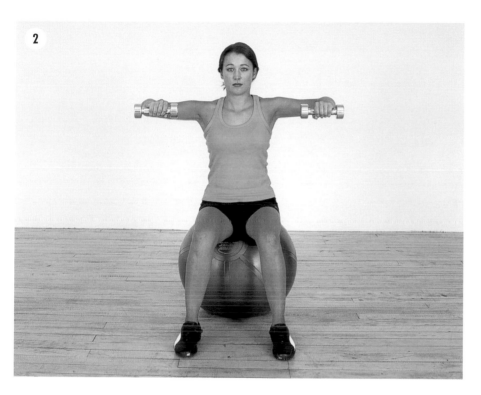

2

- Breathe out as you raise the weights until your hands, forearms, upper arms and elbows are all level with your shoulders, yet still locked at right angles.

- This is a smooth, sweeping movement. There should be no independent movement of the wrist, forearm, upper arm or head.
- Do 25 repetitions (or until fatigued).

- Allow your knees to turn outwards or inwards.
- Allow the weights to come down by picking up speed.

SEATED BICEP CURL

Strengthens the arms

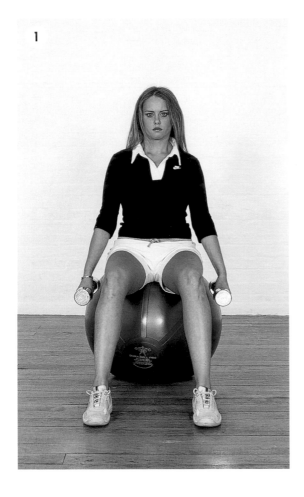

1

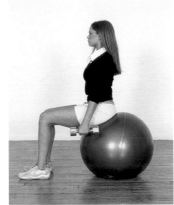

- Assume the correct seated position on the Swiss ball (see page 112).
- Sit on the ball with a dumbbell in each hand, with your arms hanging by the sides of your thighs.
- Tuck in your stomach.
- Soften your neck.
- Hold the weights down by your side, with your palms facing inwards.
- Remember that your arm is a hinge; you should only work the elbow and below. During this exercise, your upper arms should remain tucked into your sides at all times.

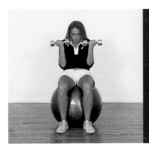

DON'T:
- Cut down the range of movement.
- Allow the weights to come down by picking up speed.

WHAT AM I DOING?

Strengthening the elbow flexors – the biceps. The secondary benefit is to stretch out the deltoids and tricep muscles from the previous exercises.

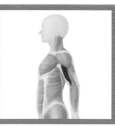

2

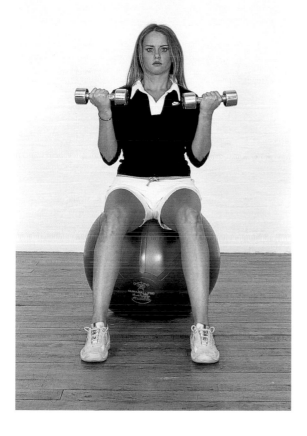

- Breathe out as you curl the weights towards your shoulders. At the end of the movement your palms should face your shoulders.
- Breathe in as you lower your arms until they are fully extended, and uncurl the weights.
- Do 25 repetitions (or until fatigued).

- Allow either of your knees to turn inwards or outwards.
- Allow your arms to swing behind you when you come down.

- Swing your arms on the way up.
- Thrust your arms into position.

LYING TRICEP EXTENSION

Strengthens the backs of the arms.

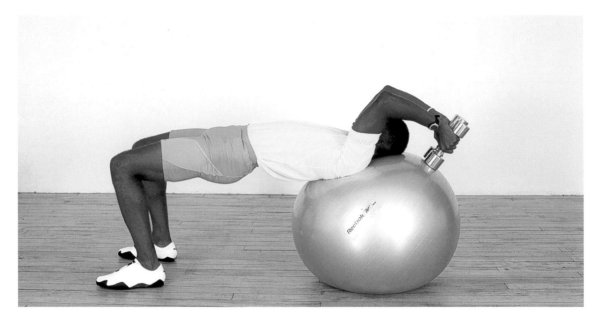

- Sit in the stabilized position with a dumbbell at each side (see page 112).
- Place the dumbbells on your thighs by your stomach.
- Walk yourself forward into the recline position as previously instructed (see page 113).
- Place your hands above your shoulders, and extend your arms.
- The dumbbells are now above the centre of your chest.

- Bring them further back so that the insides of your elbows are approximately level with your chin, and the top of your fist (your top knuckle) is above your forehead. The angle of your arm should now be challenged by gravity. You should feel tension in your triceps. Maintain this angle.
- Bend your elbows behind you. To make sure that you don't hit yourself on the crown of your head with the dumbbells, let your hands fall about 3 in (7.5 cm) apart.

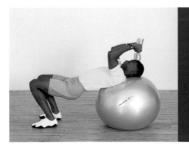

DON'T:
- Let your hips sag.
- Hold the weights directly above your forehead.

WHAT AM I DOING?

Strengthening the triceps, at the back of the upper arms. The secondary benefit is that you stretch the biceps from the previous exercises.

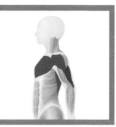

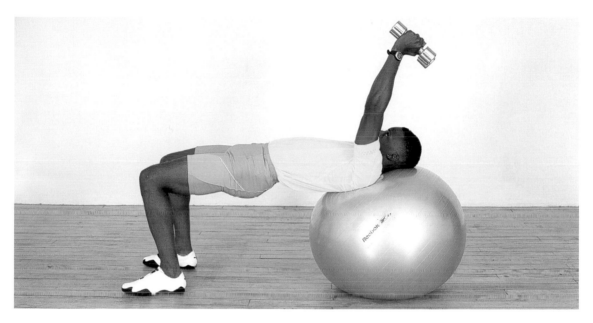

- Breathe out while you extend your arms back to the straight position. Your fists should be above the line of your forehead.
- Breathe in as you bend your elbows behind you again.
- When you have completed 25 repetitions (or until fatigued) bend your elbows and bring down your arms to your sides, returning the dumbbell to the middle of your chest.
- Lower your hips while lifting your head so that the back of your buttocks and lower back rests on the ball. Place the weights on floor, and walk yourself back into the upright seated position.
- Rest.

- **Have your heels under your buttocks.**
- **Let the weight pick up speed.**

9

TRICEP CHAIR DIP

Strengthens the back of the arms and the shoulders

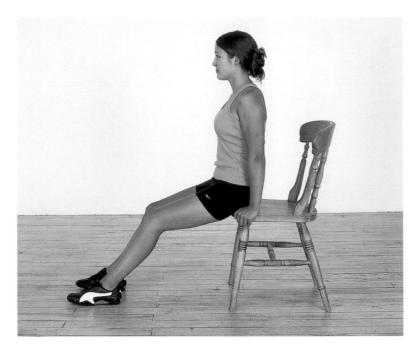

- This exercise can be done at home on a chair, as long as you have adequate room for your forearms and the chair doesn't have side bolsters. Choose a chair that is sturdy, and which allows you to place both feet firmly on the floor.
- Sit on the chair with your hands grasping the edges

by the sides of your thighs. Your wrists should be facing outwards, and not at an angle.
- Shift your buttocks until you are sitting just off the edge of the chair, with your knees bent at 90 degrees. Your feet should be flat on the floor.

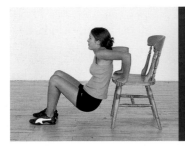

DON'T:
- Move your bottom and back more than an inch from the edge of the chair.
- Sit your weight down — lower it.

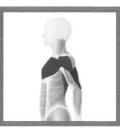

WHAT AM I DOING?

Strengthening the triceps (on the back of the upper arm) the pectoralus major muscles of the chest and the anterior fibres of the deltoids on the shoulder. The secondary benefit is that you stretch and clean the pectorals and latissimus dorsi (back muscle) from the previous exercises.

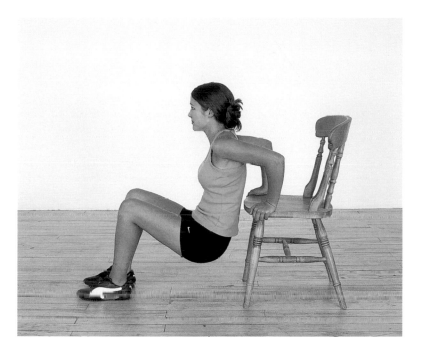

- Lower yourself off the chair by bending your elbows until the edge of the chair is level with your mid to lower back. Use only your arms to achieve this.
- Straighten your arms to push yourself back up on the chair.

- Repeat the movement.
- Do 25 repetitions (or until fatigued) without sitting back on the chair.

- Push up from the hips, thighs or legs.
- Let your shoulder and ears touch each other.

10

HALF PRESS-UP
Strengthens the chest, arms and shoulders

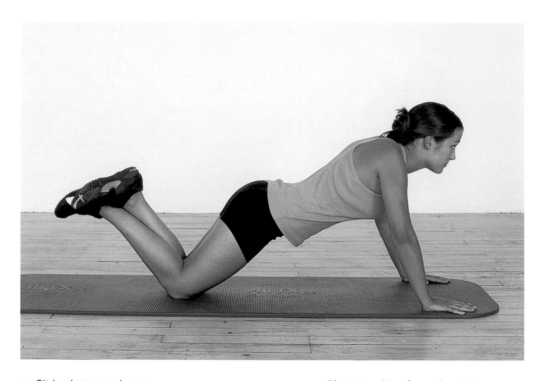

- Sit back on your knees.
- Walk your hands forward until your body is on all fours.
- Move your knees slightly apart and lock your feet.

- Move your hips forward and down.
- Your head, back and both legs should be in a straight line.

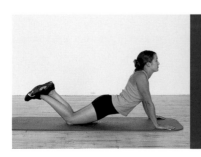

DON'T:
- Push up from your bottom.
- Arch your back.

WHAT AM I DOING?

Strengthening the pectoral muscles, the deltoids, the triceps and a whole host of other muscles, including the abdominal muscles and gluteal muscles of the hips and buttocks.

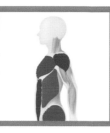

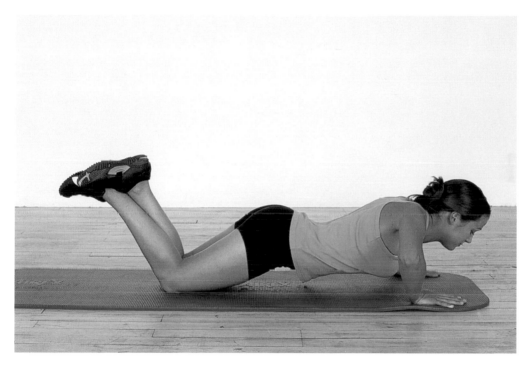

- Take your hands out slightly wider.
- Breathe in as you dip down.
- Breathe out as you go up.

- There should be no independent movement of the torso. The movement is generated by your arms.
- Do 25 repetitions (or until fatigued).

- **Let your stomach sag — remember, tight abs!**

11

FULL PRESS-UP

Strengthens the chest, shoulders, arms, back, stomach and thighs

Bodydoctor

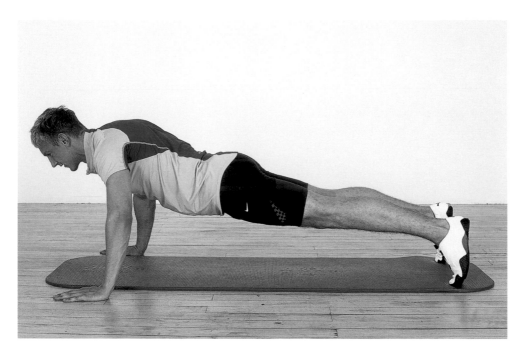

- Start from the basic half press-up position, with your knees on the floor and your upper body in a straight line.
- Move your hands further forward, until they are in line with your shoulders.

- Lift your knees off the floor.
- Balance your weight on your toes.
- Keep your head, neck, back, bottom and legs in a straight line.

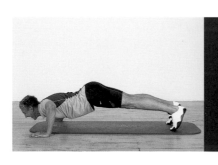

DON'T:
- Push up from your bottom.
- Arch your back.

WHAT AM I DOING?

Strengthening the pectoral muscles, the deltoids, the triceps and a range of other muscles including the abdominal muscles and gluteal muscles of the buttocks and hips.

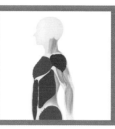

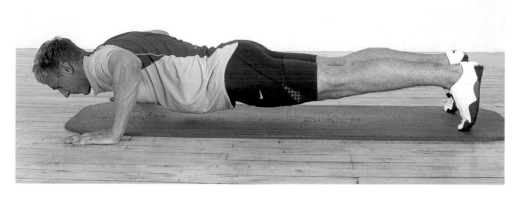

- Breathe out as you push your body up.
- Breathe in as you lower yourself to just above the floor. The movement is achieved by bending your arms at the elbows.

- Do 25 repetitions (or until fatigued). When 25 repetitions becomes easy, pause for one minute then do a repeat set.

- Allow your knees to touch the floor.
- Let your stomach sag – remember, tight abs!

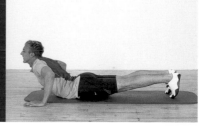

Bodydoctor®

LOWER BODY ROUTINE

LUNGES

Strengthens the thighs, buttocks, calves and hamstrings

Bodydoctor

1

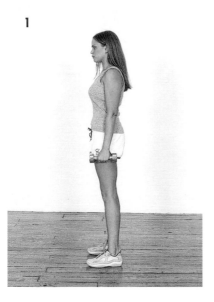

2

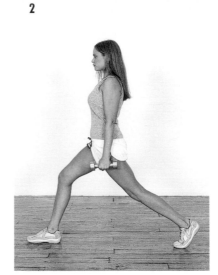

- Technique is really important in this exercise.
- Use weights that feel comfortable. Your arms should be extended by your sides, and the weights held so that your palms face inwards.
- Stand with your feet a hip-width apart. If the gym floor is wooden, a handy tip is to position your feet so that there are at least three floorboards between them (unless the floorboards are very wide).

- Pull in your stomach.
- Breathe in as you take a large step forward with your right foot, leading with your heel and planting your right foot so that your left heel comes off the floor behind you. Stop.

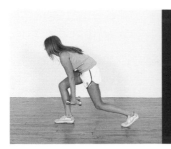

DON'T:

- Stand with your feet too wide apart.
- Stand with your feet together.
- Allow your top leg to touch the floor.

WHAT AM I DOING?

Strengthening the quadriceps on the front of the thigh, the hamstrings (on the back of the thigh), the gluteal muscles of the hips and buttocks and the calf muscles.

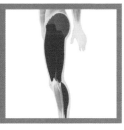

3

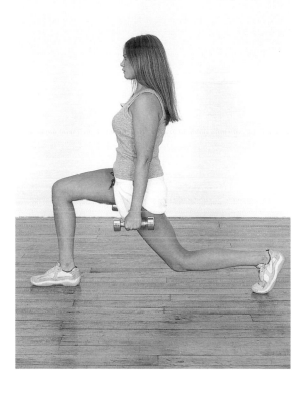

- Bend both knees simultaneously so that your left knee does not overshoot the ankle. Your left knee should now point toward the floor. Your shin should be parallel to the floor, and your left heel lifted. Stop.
- Breathe out as you push up from the right leg to the starting position in one movement.
- Take a step forward with your left leg, and repeat the exercise.
- Do 25 repetitions (or until fatigued) on each leg.

- Allow your body weight to come forward — your shoulder must remain aligned with your hips.
- Allow your back to become rounded.

13

SQUATS

Strengthens the buttocks and legs

1

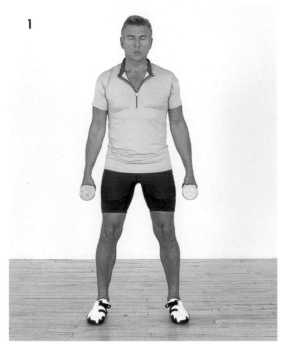

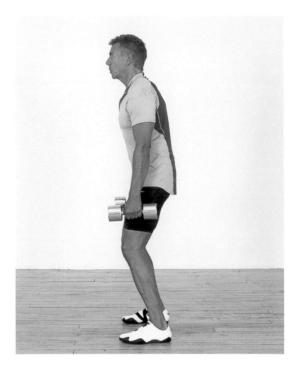

- Use weights that feel comfortable. Your arms should be extended by your sides. Hold the weights so that your palms face inwards.

- Stand with your feet level, but positioned so that they are slightly wider than your shoulders.

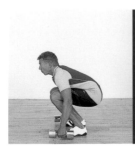

DON'T:

- Lean forward from the waist.
- Round your shoulders.
- Try to keep your back completely straight.

WHAT AM I DOING?

Strengthening the quadriceps on the front of the thigh, the gluteus medius muscle on the side of the hip, the gluteus maximus muscles of the buttocks and the hamstrings (on the back of the thigh). They affect the same muscles as those used in the Lunges (see page 142) but this exercise emphasises different parts of the muscles.

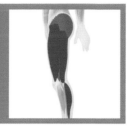

2

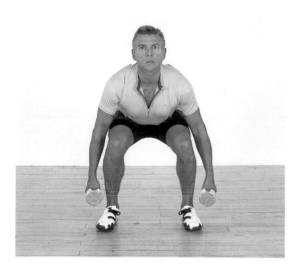

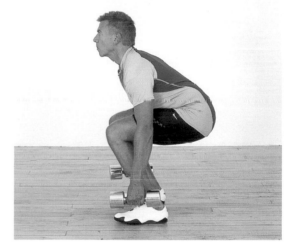

- Breathe in as you soften knees slightly; bend both knees without leaning forward too much so that your shoulders, knees and toes are all in line.
- Squat down into a semi-seated position, but not so far so that your buttocks are lower than knee height.

- Look straight ahead.
- Breathe out as you push back to a standing position, ensuring that you push through from your heels and don't just shrug your shoulders upwards.
- Do 25 repetitions (or until fatigued).

- Squat down too fast.
- Look at the floor.
- Lift your heels off the floor.

- Let the backs of your thighs make contact with the backs of your calves.

14

SIDE LEG-LIFTS
Strengthens the outer thighs and buttocks

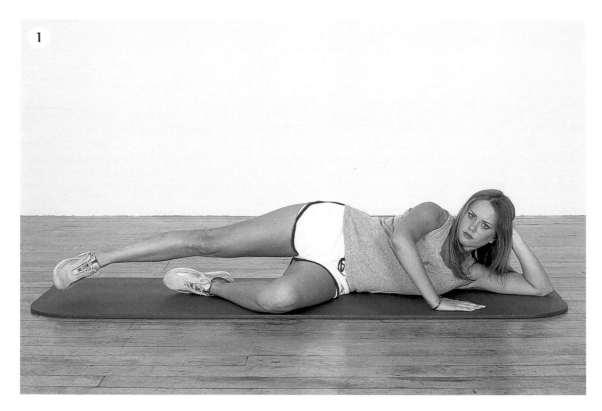

- Lie on your side with your hips stacked directly above each other.
- Support your head with your lower hand.
- Your upper hand should be on the floor in front of

your chest, acting as a stabilizer for your body, with your elbow pointing out.
- Your bottom leg should be bent.
- Your top leg should be completely straight.

DON'T:
- Allow your top hip to roll forwards or backwards.
- Try to swing your leg upwards fast.
- Let it become a continuous movement.
- Bend your leg in fast.
- Allow your top leg to touch the floor.

WHAT AM I DOING?

Strengthening the gluteal muscles (maximus and medius) of the hips and buttocks
and the hip flexor (psoas muscle).

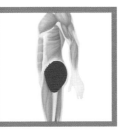

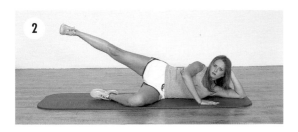

- Breathe out as you slowly lift your top leg until it is 18–24 inches (45–60 cm) above the floor. Then stop.

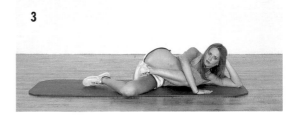

- Bend the leg (knee) slowly in towards your wrist, thus bringing your knee down towards the floor. Then stop.

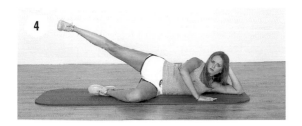

- Breathe in as you straighten the leg outwards and upwards. Then stop.

Do 25 repetitions (or until fatigued) then change sides. When you can achieve 25 repetitions, you

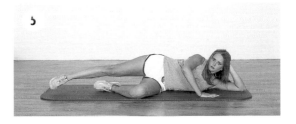

- Lower the leg to hip height. Then stop.

may want to add ankle weights – always start with the lightest weight.

Lower body routine

147

STOMACH ROUTINE

These exercises will help guys achieve a six-pack and girls attain the perfect flat stomach. The ab-flow routine must be performed in the following sequence. Do each exercise 25 times, but if this becomes too easy you'll need to increase the repetitions. When you can do 100 repetitions of each exercise in the routine, come and train me!

Bodydoctor®

AB FLOW

To maximize the results, you should keep your stomach pulled in at all times. This will help to redefine your waistline.

Using an ab-roller

The Bodydoctor says: do not try and thrust forward using your neck. You are not a woodpecker.

If you use an ab-roller for these exercises, remember that it is not there to do the work for you. A good-quality ab-roller will provide support for your neck and, if used correctly, enhance your results. Curling your chest forward from your stomach creates the momentum for the exercise. It is not achieved by pushing the ab-roller with your hands. Your hands (which should be together as if in prayer) should only rest at a right angle to the ab-roller's bar.

All you accomplish by pushing the ab-roller with your hands is to thrust the neck-rest into your neck, causing pain and possible back problems.

Your head should be placed on the centre of the neck rest and your body centralised. There should be a gap between your chin and your chest, enough to fit an apple in. If that gap closes, it means that you are thrusting forward with your head. It is not pretty, and it is definitely not clever.

Take a breath. As you breathe out, curl your chest towards your thighs. The momentum of the body will curl the body forward and back. Breathe out on the way up. Breathe in on the way back.

DON'T
- Pull and thrust with the ab-roller.
- Grip the ab-roller.

WHAT NOT TO DO WITH AN AB-ROLLER

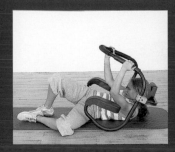 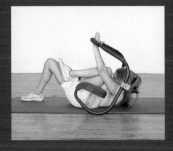 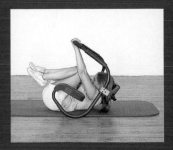

15

BASIC CRUNCHES
Strengthens the stomach muscles

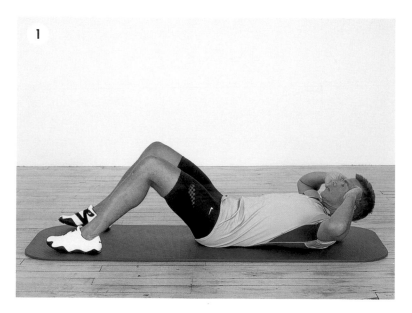

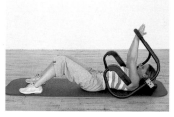

- Lay on your back, with your feet flat on the floor and hip-width apart and knees bent.
- Place your fingertips on the sides of your temples just above your ears, with your elbows open.
- Pull in your abs towards your spine and keep your head aligned.

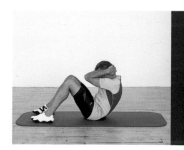

DON'T:
- Pull on the back of your head.
- Try and thrust forward by using your neck.
- Try to jerk yourself up by leading with your head.

WHAT AM I DOING?

Working the major stomach muscles – the oblique externus abdominus and oblique internus abdominus muscles, on the side and front of the torso.

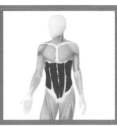

2

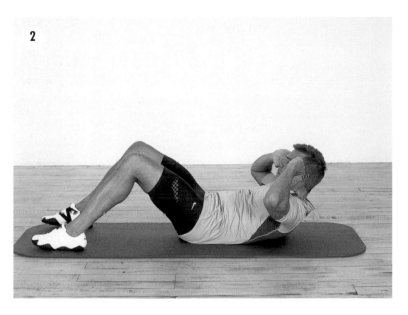

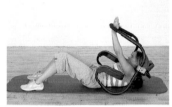

- Curl your chest 8 in (20 cm) up towards your thighs.
- Slowly lower yourself back down.

- Do 25 repetitions (or until fatigued) then return to the starting position.

16

REVERSE CURLS

Strengthens the stomach muscles

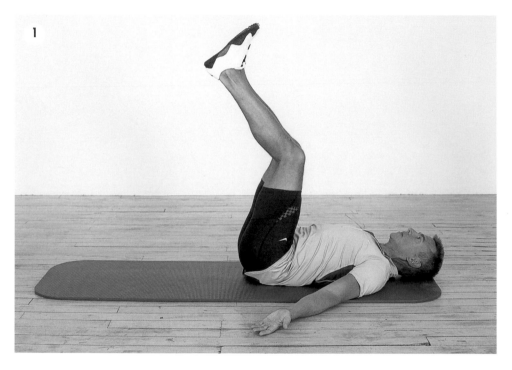

- Lay flat on the floor.
- Raise your feet and legs, so your knees and upper legs are at a right-angle to the floor.

- Place your hands on the floor beside your body, with your palms facing up.
- Suck in your lower stomach.

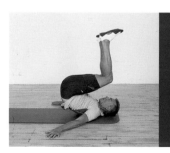

DON'T:
- Place your palms downwards, as this only encourages you to push down.
- Kick your knees to gain momentum.

WHAT AM I DOING?

Strengthening the lower fibres of the rectus abdominis (the major stomach muscle) and the hip flexors – the iliopsoas, sartorius and rectus femoris.

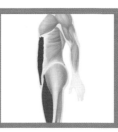

2

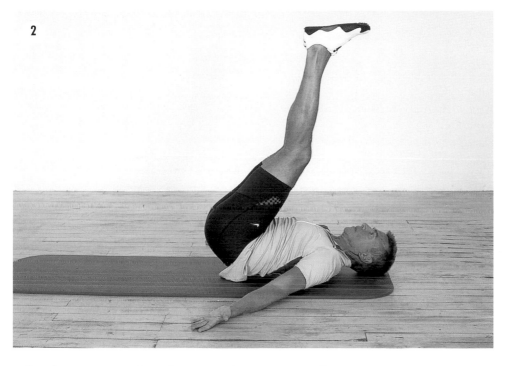

- Breathe out as you curl your knees towards your chest.
- Breathe in as you return your knees to the starting position.
- The movement should be slow.
- Do 25 repetitions (or until fatigued) then return to the starting position.

SIDE OBLIQUES

Strengthens the sides of the stomach

1

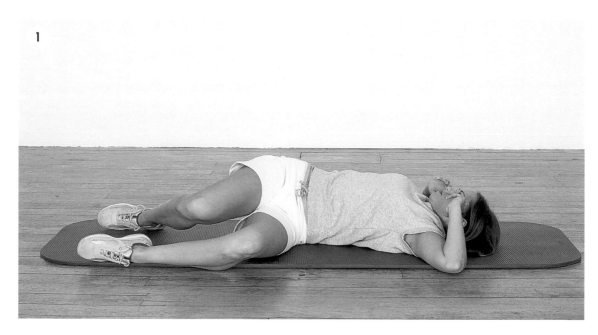

- This is a small movement, curling the chest towards the hip.
- Lay flat on floor with your knees bent. Slide your bottom to the right so that your body is kinked. Drop your knees to the left, so that your left leg is level on the floor.

- There should be a line between your forehead, hips and heels.
- Place your fingertips at the side of your head.
- Retain the gap between your chin and chest.

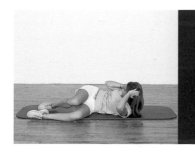

DON'T:
- Thrust forward with your head.
- Pull on the back of your neck with your hands.

WHAT AM I DOING?

Strengthening the abdominal muscles, especially the oblique internus and externus muscles on the side and front of the torso.

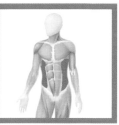

2

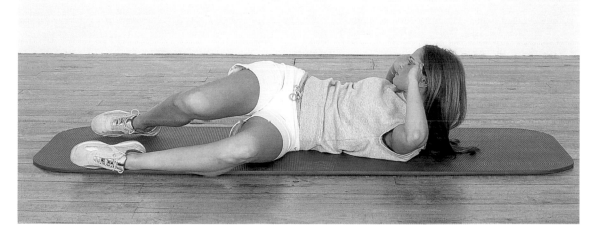

- Now curl the chest up.
- Breathe out as you curl up.
- Breathe in as you curl back.
- Do 25 repetitions (or until fatigued) then return to the starting position.
- Slide your bottom to the left.

- Now drop your knees to the right, so that your right leg is flat on the floor.
- Your heels, knees and bottom should again be aligned.
- Repeat as for the right side.

Stomach routine

155

SIDE OBLIQUES WITH
AB-ROLLER (variation)

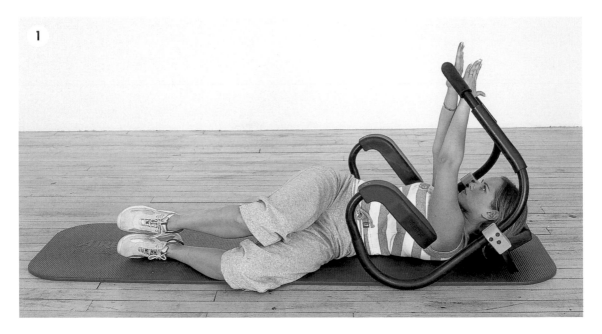

1

- Place your head on the centre of the neck rest.
- Centralize your body.
- Check that there is a gap between your chin and your chest.
- Rest your hands on the bar in the prayer position (see page 149).

- Suck in your stomach.
- Move your bottom slightly to the right.
- Drop your left knee to the side.
- Your heels, knees and hips should be aligned.

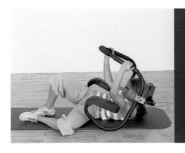

DON'T:
- Let one shoulder be higher than the other.
- Have your head facing to the side.

WHAT AM I DOING?

Strengthening the abdominal muscles, especially the oblique internus and externus muscles on the side and front of the torso.

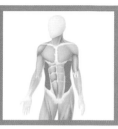

2

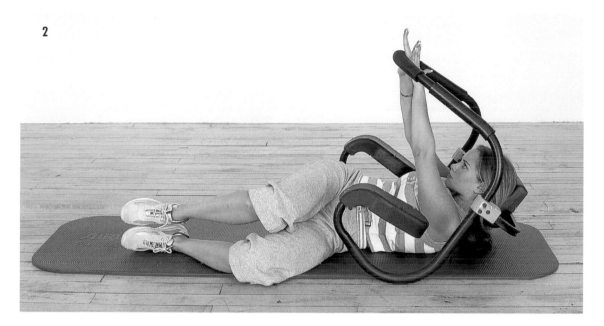

- Move your hands from the praying position. The palm of your right hand should be placed flat on the bar, keeping your right arm straight. The left arm should stretch over the top, with the palm of your left hand flattened. This pulls the left shoulder up and keeps the right shoulder down, so your body is square to the floor.
- Breathe out as you move your chest forward.
- Breathe in as you move back.
- Do 25 repetitions (or until fatigued) then return to the starting position.

- **Try to create upward momentum with your head.**
- **Pull or push on the bar with your hands.**

18A

CLIMB THE LEGS

Strengthens the stomach muscles

Bodydoctor

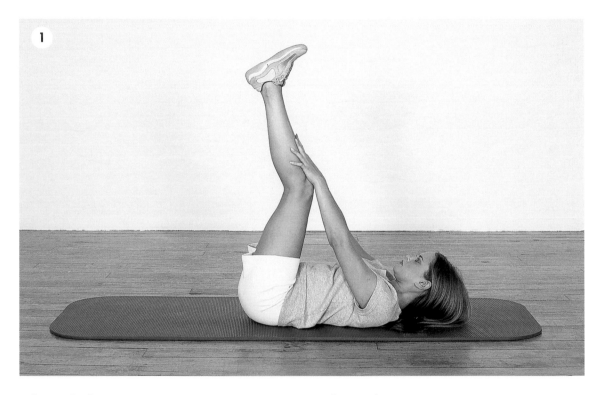

- Lay on the floor.
- Lift your legs above your hips.
- Place your hands on your shins, keeping your elbows soft.
- Raise your shoulders an inch from the floor.

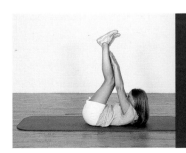

DON'T:

- Lock your elbows out.
- Create momentum by stretching your arms.
- Create momentum by jerking your head.

WHAT AM I DOING?

Strengthening the lower abdominal muscles – the rectus abdominis (the major stomach muscle), the externus and internus obliques (on the side and front of the torso) and the hip flexors.

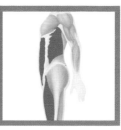

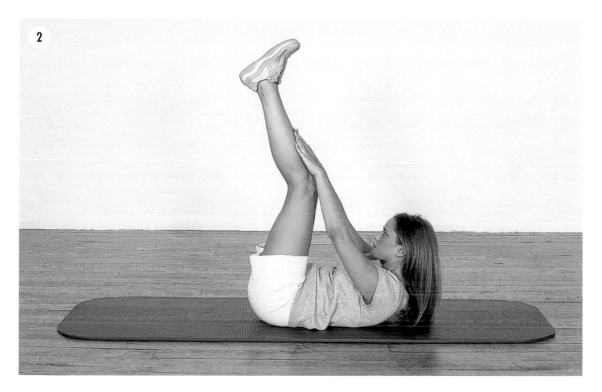

2

- Breathe out as you crunch up, moving your arms up your shins. The movement should come from your torso pushing your arms up your legs.

- Breathe in as you return to the starting position.
- Do 25 repetitions (or until fatigued).

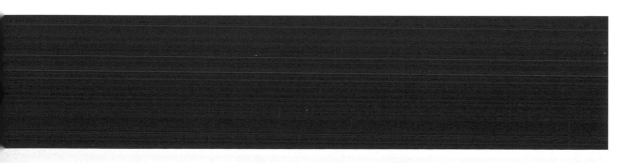

CLIMB THE LEGS WITH AB-ROLLER (variation)

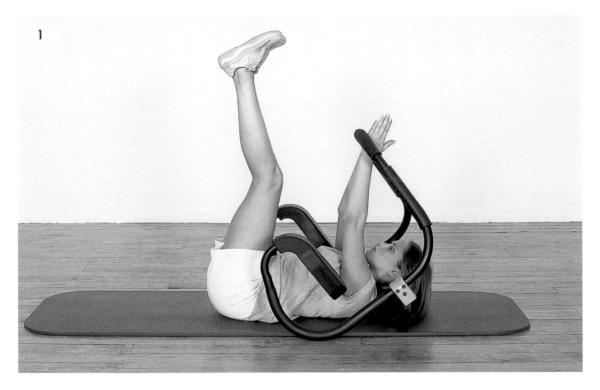

1

- Place your head on the centre of the neck rest.
- Centralize your body.
- Check that there is a gap between your chin and your chest.

- Rest your hands on the bar in prayer position (see page 149).
- Raise your legs straight up so that your body is at right angles.

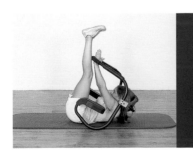

DON'T:
- Lock your elbows out.
- Curl your legs in towards the bar.

WHAT AM I DOING?

Strengthening the lower abdominal muscles – the rectus abdominis (the major stomach muscle), the externus and internus obliques (on the side and front of the torso) and the hip flexors.

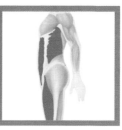

2

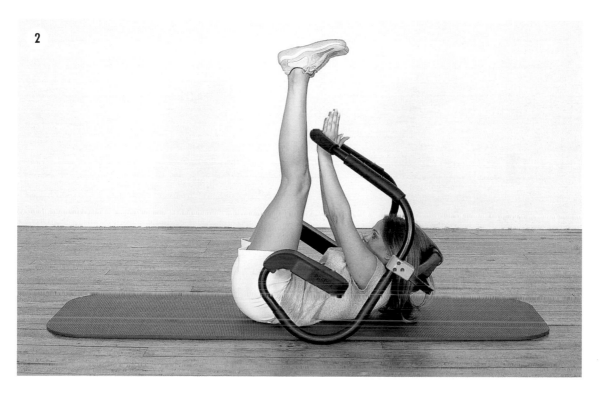

- Suck in your stomach.
- Breathe out as you crunch up, moving your arms up your shins.

- Breathe in as you return to the starting position.
- Do 25 repetitions (or until fatigued).

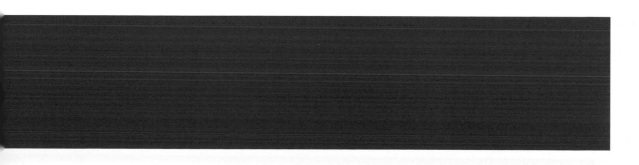

19

ELEVATED CRUNCHES WITH AB-ROLLER

Strengthens the stomach muscles

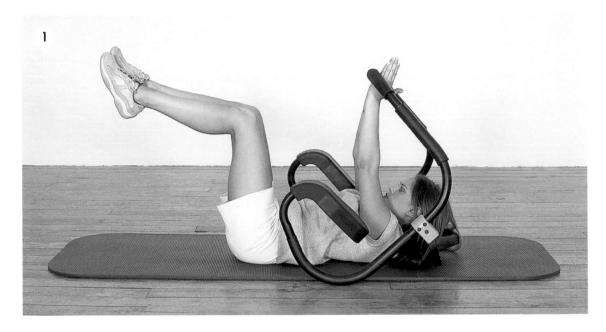

1

- Place your head on the centre of the neck rest.
- Centralize your body.
- Check that there is a gap between your chin and your chest.

- Rest your hands on the bar in prayer position (see page 149).
- Lift your legs in the air with your knees bent at a right angle. Keep your feet together.

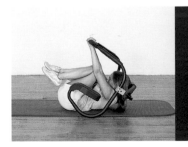

DON'T:

- Allow your knees to move further forward than your hips, because this stresses the lower back.
- Bring your knees into your arms.

WHAT AM I DOING?

Strengthening the lower abdominal muscles – the rectus abdominis, the major stomach muscles, the externus and internus obliques on the front and side of the torso and the hip flexors.

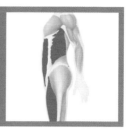

2

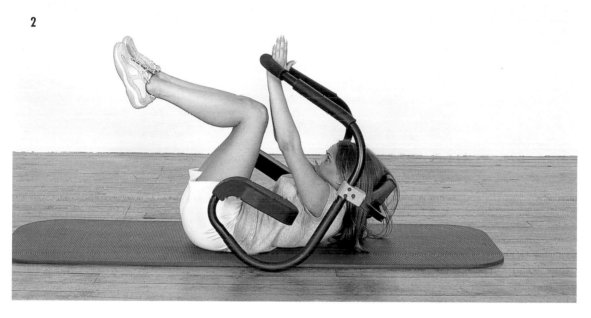

- Suck in your stomach.
- Take a breath.
- Breathe out on way up.

- Breathe in on way down.
- Do 25 repetitions (or until fatigued).

20

ALTERNATING KNEE-IN CRUNCH WITH AB-ROLLER

Strengthens the stomach muscles

1

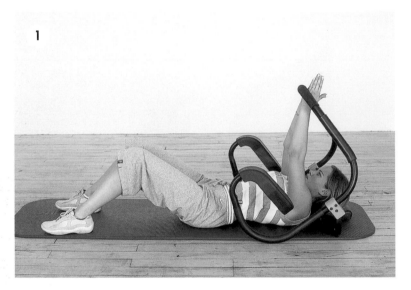

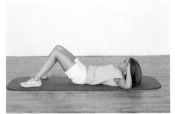

- Place your head on the centre of the neck rest.
- Centralize your body.
- Check that there is a gap between your chin and your chest.

- Rest your hands on the bar in the prayer position (see page 149).
- Keep your feet flat on the floor and bend your knees.

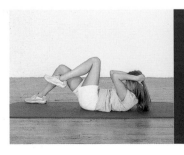

DON'T:
- Pull on the back of your head.
- Thrust forward by using your neck.
- Try to jerk up by leading with your head.

WHAT AM I DOING?

Working the major stomach muscles, or rectus abdominis; the oblique muscles (internal and external). By bringing up your knee towards your head you are using the psoas and rectus femoris (hip flexor) muscles.

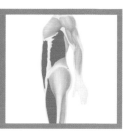

2

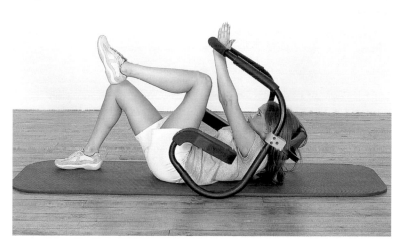

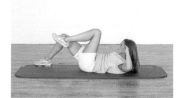

- Pull in your stomach.
- Take a breath.
- Breathe out as you crunch up, simultaneously moving one knee in to meet the forearm.

- Breathe in as you move back, allowing your knee to resume the starting position with the foot flat on the floor.
- Do 25 repetitions (or until fatigued).

Stomach routine

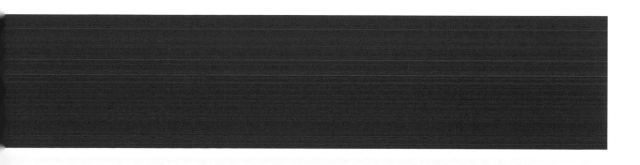

21

BICYCLE WITH AB-ROLLER

Strengthens the stomach muscles

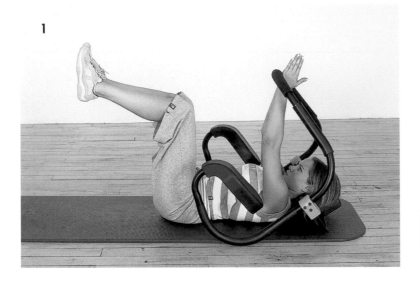

1

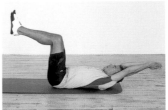

- Lie on your back with your legs bent.
- Place your head on the centre of the neck rest.
- Centralize your body.
- Check there is a gap between your chin and your chest.

- Rest your hands on the bar in a prayer position.
- Lift your legs in the air with your knees bent at a right angle.
- Keep your feet together.
- Tuck in your stomach.

DON'T:
- Allow your knees to move further forward than your hips when in the starting position as this stresses the lower back.

Bodydoctor

WHAT AM I DOING?

Working the major stomach muscles, or rectus abdominis; the oblique muscles (internal and external). By bringing up your knee towards your head you are using the psoas and rectus femoris (hip flexor) muscles.

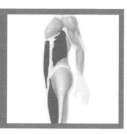

2

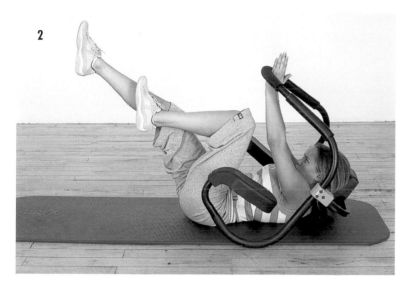

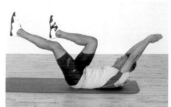

- As you curl your chest towards your thighs, exhaling, bring one knee in towards your forearms and extend one leg out to an almost straight leg position.
- Come back to the middle with your knees above your hips and your shoulder blades back on the floor.
- Repeat by changing legs.
- Start with as many pairs (right leg, left leg) as you can, building up to 25 pairs.

22

PRAYERS

Strengthens the stomach muscles

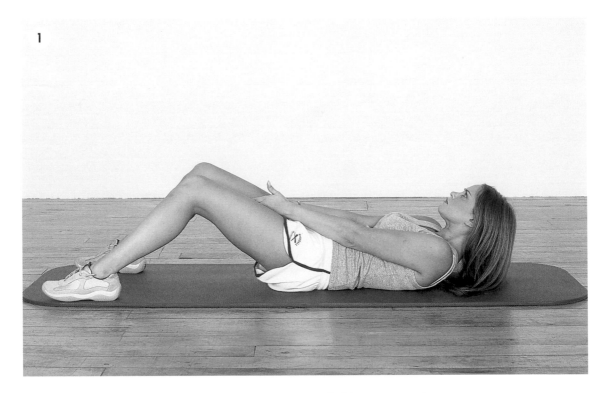

1

- Lay on your back.
- Bend your knees, keeping your feet slightly apart.
- Stretch arms above head, with both hands in the prayer position.

- Pull in your stomach.
- Bring down your hands between your legs, pulling your body up off your shoulder blades. Your hands should reach out in a stretch position. This is your starting position.

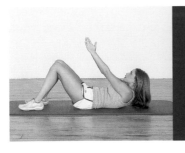

DON'T:
- Start with soft elbows and then stretch out with your hands, using them to propel your body forwards.

WHAT AM I DOING?

The Bodydoctor says:

Knackering yourself. Burning off the last remains of resistance from the adipose army. Exhausting the muscle fibres from the previous exercises.

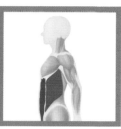

2

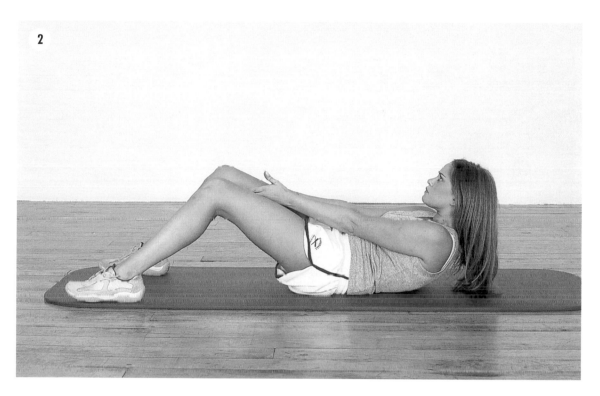

- Breathe out. As you crunch forwards, your hands are pushed forward (still in prayer position) between your legs.
- Breathe in as you move slowly back to the starting position.
- The trajectory of your hands should remain low.
- Do 25 repetitions (or until fatigued).

23

LOWER BACK EXTENSION

Strengthens the lower back muscles and buttocks

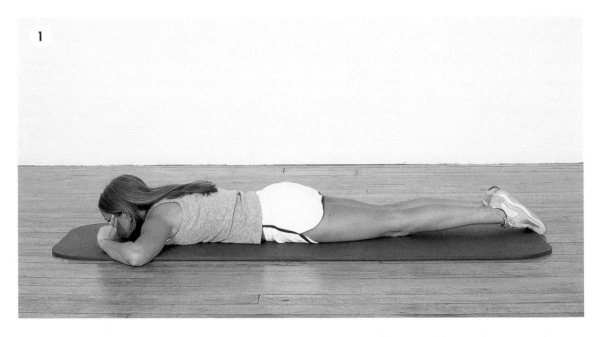

1

- Lay flat on your front.
- Look straight ahead, resting your chin on the floor.
- Place your fingertips at your temples.

- Place your feet and ankles together, so your legs are in a straight line.

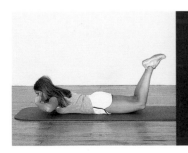

DON'T:
- Jerk up fast.
- Let your legs bend at the knee.

WHAT AM I DOING?

Strengthening the erector spinae muscles (attached to the vertebrae), the hamstring muscles and the gluteal muscles of the buttocks and the quadratus lumborum. The secondary effect is to stretch the abdominal muscles that you've worked previously. It also stretches the psoas muscle, or hip flexor.

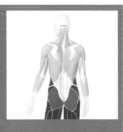

2

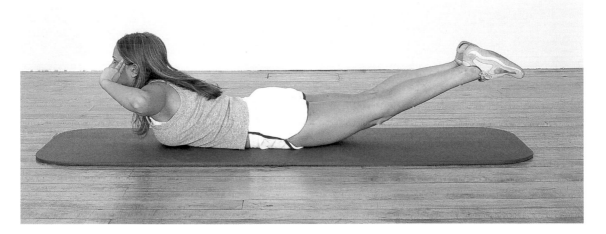

- Breathe out as you slowly lift up your legs (in a straight line) from just above your knees, simultaneously raising your chest. Your lower torso and upper thighs should remain on the floor.
- Breathe in as you return to the starting position.

Your chin and toes should touch the floor at the same time.
- This is a slow, fluid movement.
- Do 25 repetitions (or until fatigued).

THREE STRETCHES TO CLEAN THE ABDOMINAL AND LOWER BACK MUSCLES

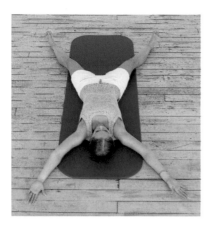

- I call this the 'X stretch'.
- Lay on your back, with your arms and legs extended out to the sides to make the shape of a big cross. Stretch your fingertips away from you, and stretch your legs downwards by pushing down from your heels. Stretch yourself out from all four points.
- Hold the stretch and breathe normally.

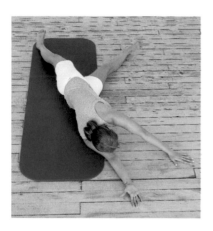

- Start by lying on the floor on your back in the 'X stretch'. Inhale deeply.
- As you exhale, keep your left arm straight and twist your body over to your right side so you get a twist at the waist. Keep both feet and your right arm anchored to the floor.
- Inhale as you stretch the fingertips of your left hand away from you, push down from your left and right heels, and stretch the fingertips of your right hand. Hold the position, breathing normally.
- Inhale as you relax and lay back on the floor.
- Repeat on the other side.

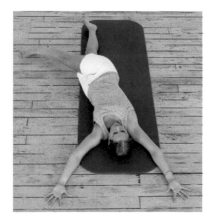

- Lie on your back in the 'X stretch' (see above) and inhale.
- Extend your right leg over your right thigh, and push your left heel down.
- Stretch both hands and feet away from your body. Hold the stretch and breathe normally.
- Inhale as you return to the cross position.
- Repeat with the left leg.

CARDIOVASCULAR

TRAINING — FAT BURNING AND AEROBIC CONDITIONING

Bodydoctor®

Finish the exercise programme with 15–45 minutes' cardiovascular work at a reasonable intensity i.e., 65–75 per cent of your maximum heart rate (see page 16) – or up to 75–80 per cent if you are already very fit and do not have any excess body fat that you want to burn – on a step machine, rowing machine, stationary bike or treadmill in the gym (see Warming up page 80 to refresh your technique).

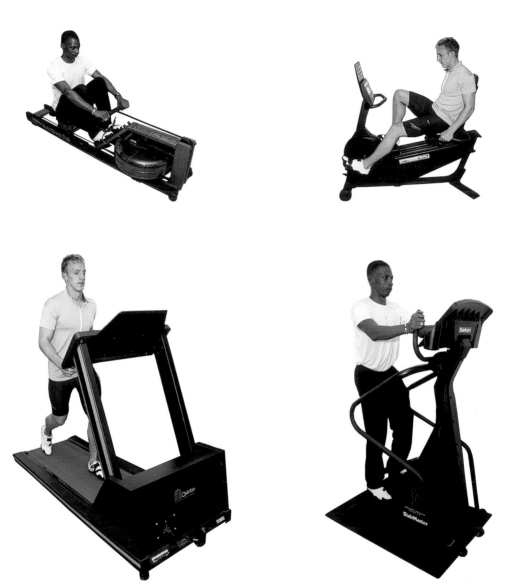

Outdoor cardio

As an alternative or supplement to the gym-based cardiovascular, here are the additions to power walking and jogging. Again, the constant factor should be working at a sustainable heart rate of 65–75 per cent to burn fat, or up to 85 per cent if you want to make considerable gains to your cardiovascular fitness.

How to begin

If you have never exercised before, for the first six weeks simply walk for 10 to 20 minutes at a comfortable pace that leaves you sweaty. If you are not sweaty then, you're not working hard enough. Keep track of how far you travel in the time. Look out for landmarks, but remember that you don't want to see the same ones every time. Try to find a new landmark that's further on from the previous one. You should be walking further and further each time. If you are generally fit, start out with a 45-minute walk, building up to a 15-minute run. Experienced keep-fit trainers should start with a 30-minute run.

The importance of variety

Cardiovascular activity can, I am afraid, be boring. Very few of us really enjoy a 5-mile run. The best way to keep up your enthusiasm is to inject a bit of variety into your training. Here are some of the training modules that Steve Marshall (see page 62) used at England Under-21 rugby training camps. And you don't need to be a towering beefcake to do them – everyone can benefit.

Why not try shuttles?

Place a marker, which can be a tracksuit jacket or a large stick, 25 metres from where you intend to start running. Five metres equals approximately five large strides for an average adult. Place another marker 20 strides on from that and another marker 20 strides on again.

After your warm-up, start jogging to the first marker and then walk back to the starting position. Jog to the second marker and walk back to the start. Jog to the third marker and walk back to the beginning. Repeat five times. Build up to 10 times. When this becomes easy, upgrade to running and jogging.

After another week lengthen the distance between the markers. Always work yourself to the hardest you possibly can, when you are trying to obtain optimum fitness.

What about some Fartlek runs?

This exercise simply requires you to walk, then jog and then stride. Simple, huh?

You should walk at a pace that is faster than you would use to walk down to the shops, have a sweat on and feel a lot warmer, then you should jog slowly at a pace you feel comfortable with and then stride at a faster pace than the jog. As you can see, you are building the pace up. Initially spend one minute on each section; that is, walking, jogging, striding. Keep repeating the challenge. When you can comfortably jog for the second portion, push up to a run. Within six weeks you should manage to lengthen the time that you spend on each portion to five minutes. So that's five minutes walking, jogging and striding! And you must repeat this as soon as you feel comfortable striding! As soon as you feel comfortable striding, you should push yourself harder – as this will achieve maximum results.

What about Quadrant runs?

This exercise requires a football pitch or rugby ground.

Quite simply, you begin by walking the length of the pitch, running the diagonal and sprinting the width. You should aim to spend 20–30 minutes working out this way. You can then build up to walking the length of the pitch, jogging the diagonal, sprinting the width and jogging the other diagonal. After a few weeks you should be able to run further, so jog the diagonal of the pitch and sprint the width. Vary your workout to suit your progress.

What about skipping?

Boxers and young children in the school playground make this look incredibly easy, but skipping is an exceptional cardio workout. It tones the muscles of the upper body and the lower body, defines the abdominal muscles and helps reduce cellulite. Some experts reckon that 10 minutes of skipping is equivalent to 30 minutes of running at a reasonably fast pace. It burns around 12 calories per minute for an 11-stone person.

You need a good rope. A nylon rope requires you to work hard to turn it fast. A leather rope may turn easier but is heavier, so it works the muscles more. Stand on the centre of the rope and lift up the handles. If the rope is the right length, the handles should meet your armpits. Because you will be jumping up and down, it is very important that you wear trainers with good shock absorbency. You should also jump on softer surfaces – concrete can be too hard.

Start slowly. Jump for a minute or two, then rest for a similar period. Stretch your calves. Aim to jump 60–70 times in one minute. Even

jumping a couple of inches off the ground is a great workout. Turn the rope with your wrists and forearms – not the shoulders. Build up the time you skip for, but always take a short rest to stretch the calves.

What about cycling?

Start with a 15–20-minute bicycle ride. You should feel comfortable, and not too out of breath. Build up to cycling for an hour.

Cycling brings its own dangers, though. If you cycle at night, make sure you have proper reflective clothing so that you can see and be seen, and wear a safety helmet at all times.

Planning

You cannot rush what you want to do. Do not expect to achieve a four-minute mile if you have never run before. Be realistic! In the first six weeks you want to condition your body to get it used to doing cardiovascular work. It will take time to increase your stamina and flexibility. After six weeks, you should increase the intensity and time devoted to your training. And after 12 weeks, start to keep records of your times and distances. This will help motivate you, especially if you constantly aim to beat the best time or distance. But you will have your off-days too, when your times go awry. If you're having an off day, don't worry; everyone has bad days. Just put it to the back of your mind and plan to work harder the next day.

Always allow yourself rest days – I recommend a minimum of two rest days a week on which you do not train. And I do mean rest. Don't be tempted to go for a half-hour walk around the block. It will not speed up results, and could actually lead to injuries. This is because the body needs time to recuperate after exercising. Sleep is the biggest component of fitness. When you sleep, you recuperate. Paula Radcliffe will sleep for a minimum of 11 hours a day, and usually has two hours extra in the afternoons.

Always try to get yourself eight hours of unbroken sleep each night.

Cool down

You may think that as soon as you finish your jog, you can just jump in the car to drive home or jump in a shower! Well, you're wrong: cooling down is just as important as warming up. It helps to release the waste products that build up during exercise, and will help your muscles return to their normal lengths. You cool down exactly the same way that you warm up, but with less intensity.

FLEXIBILITY EXERCISES

Strong as oaks, flexible as reeds.

FLEXIBILITY EXERCISES: THE BENEFITS

The exercises:

1) Reduce muscle ache.

2) Increase co-ordination.

3) Increase the flow of lubricating fluid around the joints, increasing the range of movement.

4) Increase the circulation of the blood.

5) Decrease scar tissue – when you stretch, scar tissue is broken.

6) Stretch the connective tissue of muscle, helping it maintain its elasticity and improving flexibility.

STARTING POSITION

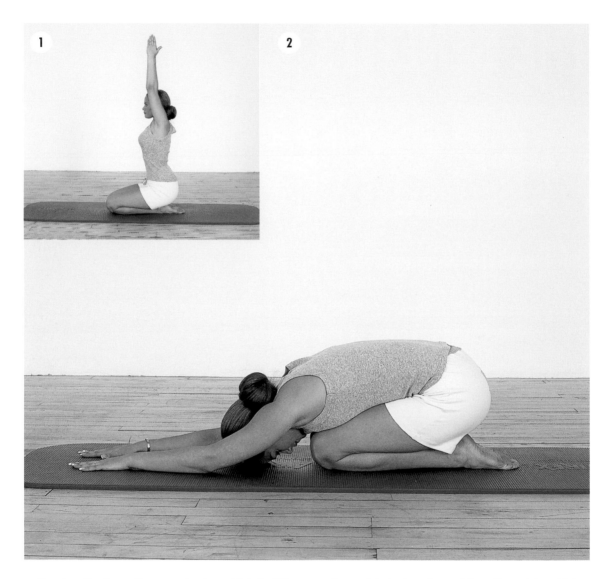

- Kneel on the floor, sit on your heels and inhale. Lift your ribcage, pull in your abdomen and stretch your spine upwards.
- Stretch your arms above your head. Stretch through into your fingertips.
- Keep your breathing slow and even.
- Increase the stretch.

- As you inhale, lean forward from the waist and let your upper body become part of your lower body.
- Let your head touch the floor and your hands stretch out in front of you, and inhale.
- As you exhale, stretch your fingers out in front of you.
- Breathe slowly, evenly and relax – everywhere.
- Breathe as you come up and get up slowly.

STRETCH 1

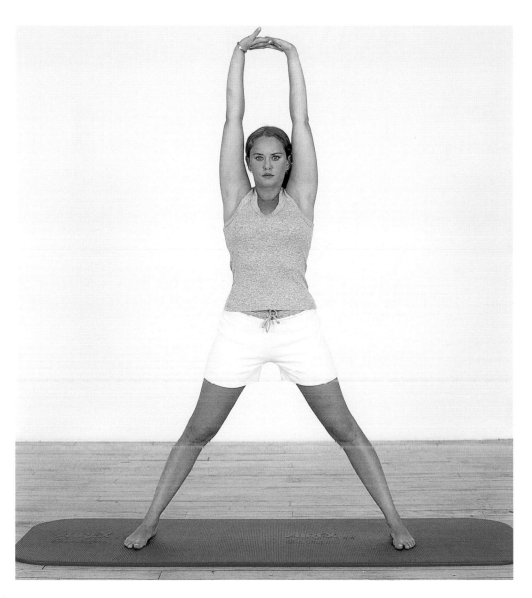

• Stand with your feet wide. Breathe in and, as you push your arms towards the ceiling, breathe out.

Interlock your fingers, turn your palms up towards the ceiling and push upwards.

STRETCH 2

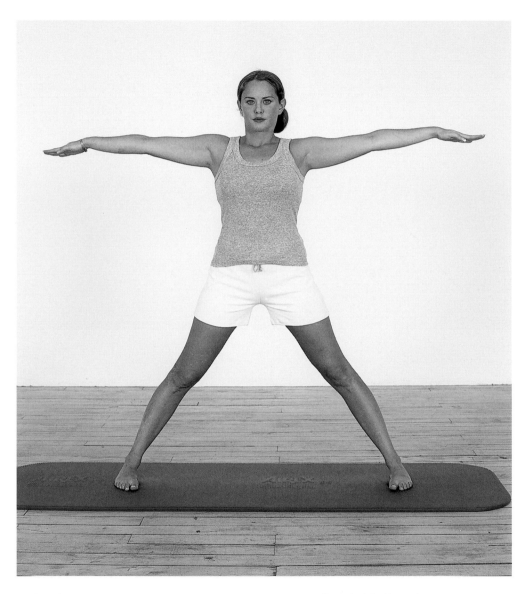

- Breathe in as your arms come up to shoulder height. Exhale as you push both arms outwards.

- Stretch right through to your fingertips.

STRETCH 3

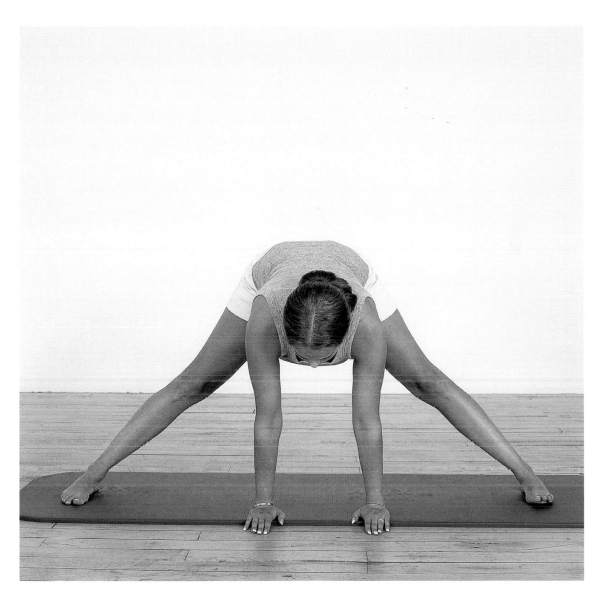

- Inhale as you bring your arms straight out in front of you.
- Breathe out and lean forward from the waist, not from the back, so your palms touch the floor. Do not round your back.
- Hold the stretch, breathing normally.

- If you cannot reach the floor, put your hands on your shins and go down as far as you can.
- Keep your thigh muscles working with your kneecaps pulled in.
- Inhale as you stand up straight.

STRETCHES 4 & 5

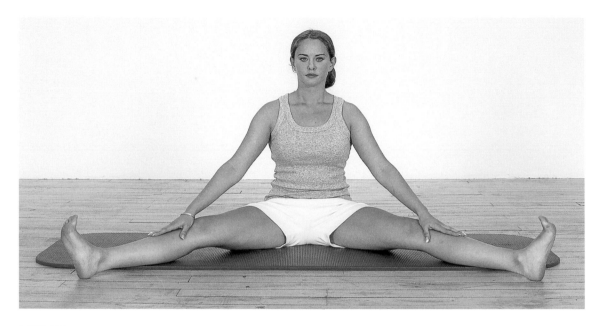

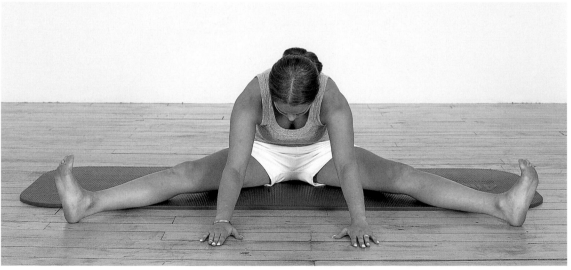

- Sit on the floor on the front of your bottom rather than your tailbone. Inhale.
- Open your legs as far as possible. Pull your toes up, pull your lower stomach in, lift your ribcage and sit tall.
- Hold the stretch.

- Exhale as you lean forward from the waist (not from your shoulders) and extend your arms in front of you.
- Hold the stretch, breathing normally.
- Inhale as you sit up straight.

STRETCH 6

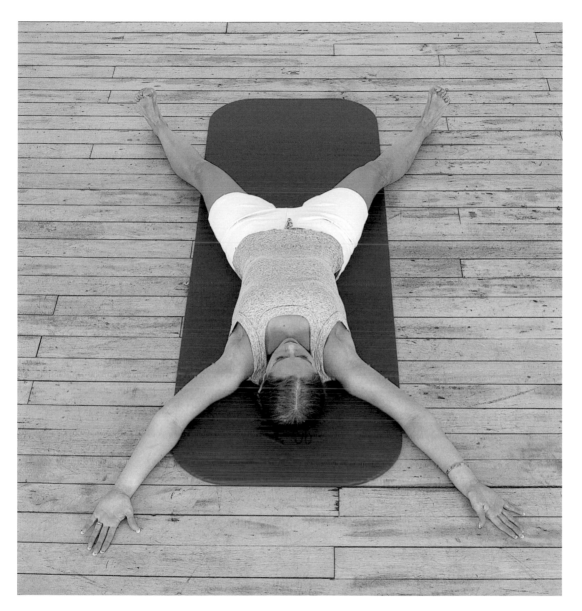

- I call this the 'X stretch'.
- Lay on your back, with your arms and legs extended out to the sides to make the shape of a big cross. Stretch your fingertips away from you, and stretch your legs downwards by pushing down from your heels. Stretch yourself out from all four points.
- Hold the stretch and breathe normally.

STRETCH 7

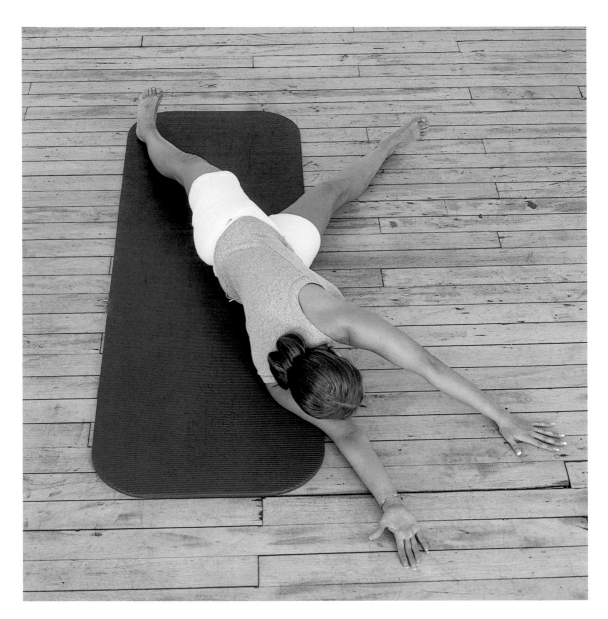

- Start by lying on the floor on your back in the 'X stretch'. Inhale deeply.
- As you exhale, keep your left arm straight and twist your body over to your right side so you get a twist at the waist. Keep both feet and your right arm anchored to the floor.

- Inhale as you stretch the fingertips of your left hand away from you, push down from your left and right heels, and stretch the fingertips of your right hand.
- Hold the position, breathing normally.
- Inhale as you relax and lay back on the floor.

STRETCH 8

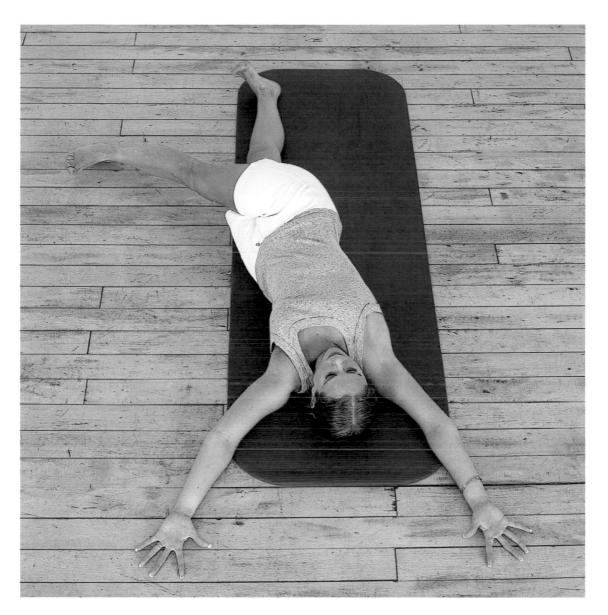

- Lie on your back in the 'X stretch' (see Stretch 6, page 185) and inhale.
- Extend your right leg over your left thigh, and push your left heel down.

- Stretch both hands and feet away from your body. Hold the stretch and breathe normally.
- Inhale as you return to the cross position.
- Repeat with the left leg.

STRETCHES 9 & 10

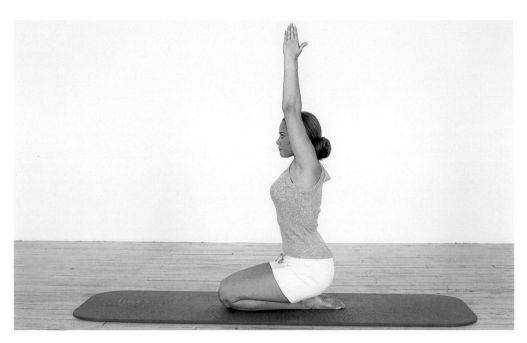

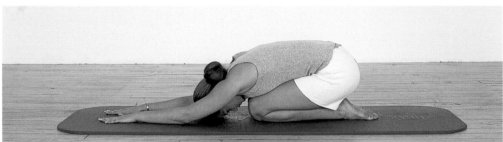

- Kneel on the floor, sit on your heels and inhale. Lift your ribcage, pull in your abdomen and stretch your spine upwards.
- Stretch your arms above your head. Stretch through into your fingertips.
- Let your neck and head relax. Imagine that your neck is an oasis of tranquillity surrounded by a maelstrom of activity.
- Increase the stretch. Reach for the sky.
- As you inhale, lean forward from the waist and let your upper body become part of your lower body.
- Let your head touch the floor and your hands stretch out in front of you, and inhale.
- As you exhale, stretch your fingers out in front of you. Let your bottom become part of your heels, let your thighs become part of your calves, let your stomach become part of your thighs, let your chest become part of your knees, let your head become part of the floor. Get that sinking feeling.
- Breathe slowly, evenly and relax – everywhere.
- Breathe as you come up and get up slowly.
- Then lie on your back in the 'X stretch' as in Stretch 6 (see page 185). Breathe slowly, and let your arms and legs come back in towards the centre.

YOUR WORKOUT
IS NOW OVER

Remember to eat some protein
within 1½ hours (see page 206).

UPPER BODY

For your convenience, here is an overview of the entire workout. Photocopy it and have it encapsulated so you can use it to remind you of the order of the exercises once you are familiar with the programme and have perfected your technique. Do the same with the Golden Rules (see page 73).

Gym

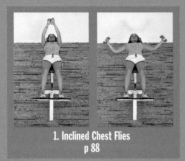

1. Inclined Chest Flies
p 88

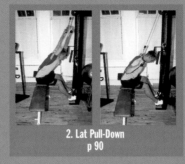

2. Lat Pull-Down
p 90

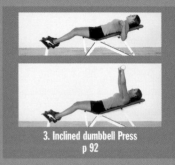

3. Inclined dumbbell Press
p 92

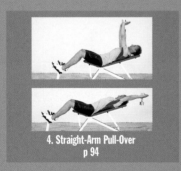

4. Straight-Arm Pull-Over
p 94

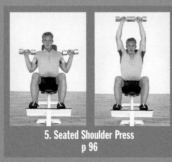

5. Seated Shoulder Press
p 96

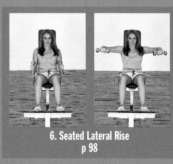

6. Seated Lateral Rise
p 98

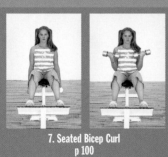

7. Seated Bicep Curl
p 100

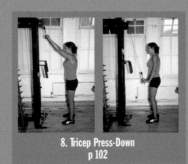

8. Tricep Press-Down
p 102

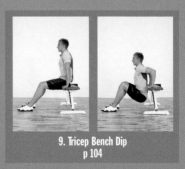

9. Tricep Bench Dip
p 104

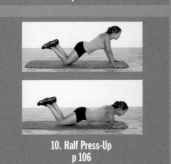

10. Half Press-Up
p 106

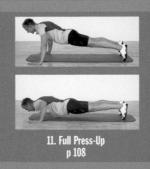

11. Full Press-Up
p 108

Home

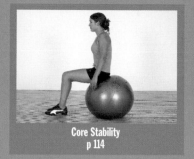
Core Stability
p 114

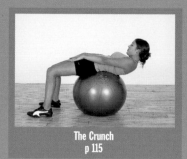
The Crunch
p 115

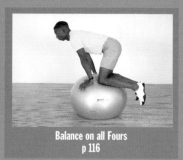
Balance on all Fours
p 116

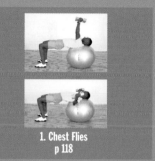
1. Chest Flies
p 118

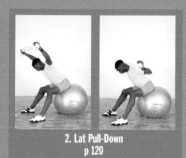
2. Lat Pull-Down
p 120

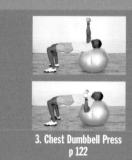
3. Chest Dumbbell Press
p 122

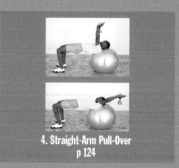
4. Straight-Arm Pull-Over
p 124

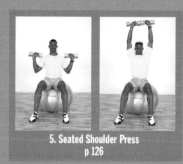
5. Seated Shoulder Press
p 126

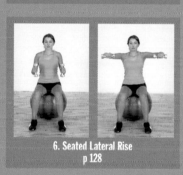
6. Seated Lateral Rise
p 128

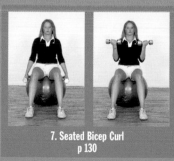
7. Seated Bicep Curl
p 130

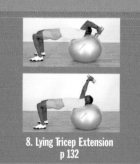
8. Lying Tricep Extension
p 132

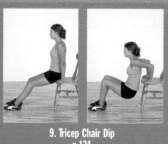
9. Tricep Chair Dip
p 134

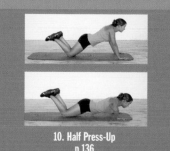
10. Half Press-Up
p 136

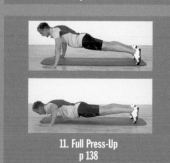

11. Full Press-Up
p 138

LOWER BODY

For your convenience, here is an overview of the entire workout. Photocopy it and have it encapsulated so you can use it to remind you of the order of the exercises once you are familiar with the programme and have perfected your technique. Do the same with the Golden Rules (see page 73).

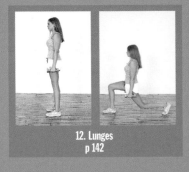

12. Lunges
p 142

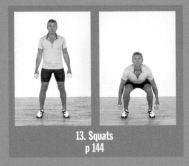

13. Squats
p 144

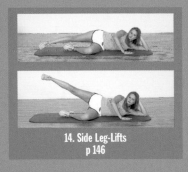

14. Side Leg-Lifts
p 146

Stomach Routine

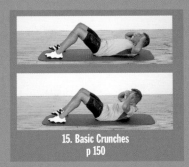

15. Basic Crunches
p 150

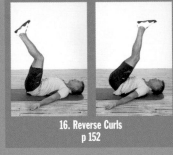

16. Reverse Curls
p 152

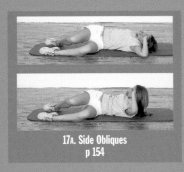

17a. Side Obliques
p 154

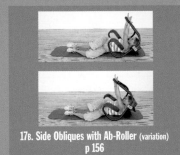

17b. Side Obliques with Ab-Roller (variation)
p 156

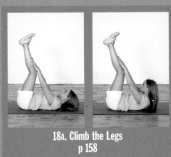

18a. Climb the Legs
p 158

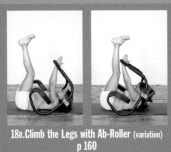

18b. Climb the Legs with Ab-Roller (variation)
p 160

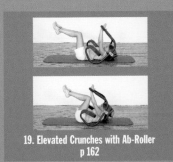

19. Elevated Crunches with Ab-Roller
p 162

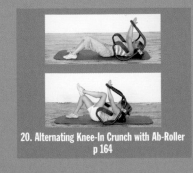

20. Alternating Knee-In Crunch with Ab-Roller
p 164

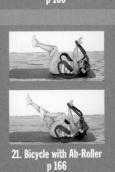

21. Bicycle with Ab-Roller
p 166

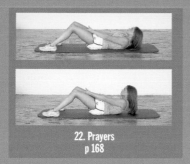

22. Prayers
p 168

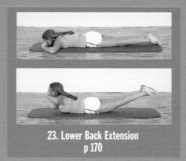

23. Lower Back Extension
p 170

Flexibility Exercises

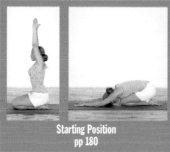

Starting Position
pp 180

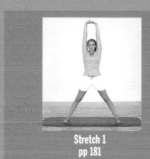

Stretch 1
pp 181

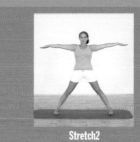

Stretch2
pp 182

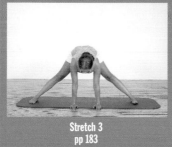

Stretch 3
pp 183

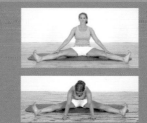
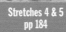

Stretches 4 & 5
pp 184

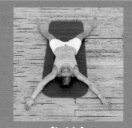

Stretch 6
pp 185

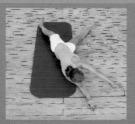

Stretch 7
pp 186

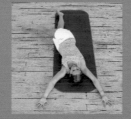

Stretch 8
pp 187

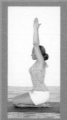
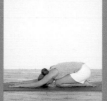

Stretches 9 & 10
pp 188

PART THREE

Nutrition with Bodydoctor Fitness

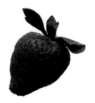

The Bodydoctor says: diets do not work. If they did, there would be one called 'The Diet', which everyone would follow, and everyone would be fit and healthy.

What to eat — and when to eat it!

We used to eat according to survival. We evolved to run after food, or escape from predators: we were the hunters or the hunted. This was exercise in its most instinctive form. We fed at naturally correct times; office lunch breaks, television schedules or trendy restaurant opening hours didn't govern our eating patterns. That's why this part of the book shows you how to eat the right foods but, just as importantly, when to eat them! (See the Golden Rules for your diet on page 216). This section gives an overview of my philosophy about nutrition, and the science behind my programme. But if you just want to get to the guts of it and choose the right foods to help you achieve your goals, skip to The Bodydoctor Nutrition Plan on page 215.

Every client has different priorities. At Bodydoctor Fitness there are new mothers who want to get back into shape after having a baby, stressed businessmen carrying too much weight and individuals recovering from serious cardiovascular problems. Some have specific health goals. Yet they each have one thing in common: a desire to improve their fitness, health and vitality, despite the barrage of confusion brought on by those shelves of nutrition books, videos and weight-loss programmes.

Some are gimmick diets, some are contradictory and some are not at all good for you. Fad diets don't work, no matter how tempting their claims may seem. Yes, you may lose weight initially, but these diets often have detrimental effects on your health, and are just not sustainable.

At Bodydoctor Fitness, we don't claim to offer a 'magic bullet' solution. We simply promote a long-term healthy eating plan, which will benefit you whatever your state of health. The programme is based on solid scientific research and the basic principle that we should eat the foods for which the body originally evolved to thrive on. Think about it.

You might not like what you're about to read. You might not agree with it, and it might fly in the face of everything that you've been told. But it's a fact: people who are seriously ill due to obesity are probably ill because for years they've been using their teeth as grave diggers. The food that they eat is populated with chemicals, hormones and pesticides.

YOU DID NOT COME FROM A CHEMICAL LAB. YOU DID NOT EVOLVE TO CONSUME CHEMICALS. ARE YOUR TEETH FOOD PROCESSORS OR GRAVE DIGGERS? IT'S MAKE-YOUR-MIND-UP TIME.

Put the right foods into your body, or you'll be in a state of decline from day one. The choice is yours. If you can't be bothered, put this book down now.

As I've said earlier, no one ever got fit and slim, trim and lovely by sitting on their bum on a couch reading about it or watching a video. Your destiny is in your hands: no one determines your shopping list when you go to the supermarket but you. No one determines your energy expenditure but you. If you're not going to do it for yourself, no one will.

Do the right thing. Read on, and do something.

What's wrong with the modern diet?

Or perhaps, more accurately, what's right with it? We may have reduced our intake of calories and fat over the past 30 years, but the incidence of obesity, heart disease, diabetes and hormonal-related cancers has risen dramatically. One in eight women are now affected by breast cancer. That rate has tripled over the past 30 years, but in 20 years time doctors predict that one in four[1] women may be affected! A 65-year-old male is now 30 per cent more likely to suffer from heart disease than he was 50 years ago[2]. Teenagers are showing signs of blocked arteries, which is a contributing factor in heart disease. Children under 10 are being diagnosed with type II diabetes[3]. Historically, this form of diabetes, caused primarily by too much sugar in the diet, was rarely seen in youngsters. There is clinical research to support the fact that nutritional status is partly responsible for every single one of these shocking statistics. In short, the modern diet is having a disastrous impact on the health of the nation.

Irresponsible food manufacturers?

In 2002, an overweight American man sued four fast-food chains because he blamed them for his obesity. The courts did not find in his favour, but it is certainly true that the modern food industry is contributing to the nation's ill-health. So what has happened to the food that we eat unthinkingly every day? Here are just some examples:

- Refined sugar is added to almost everything. On average, we each consume over 4 oz (100 g) a day, when our bodies can barely cope with more than a teaspoon (see page 199).
- Flour is refined to offer us more palatable 'white' products such as bread, cakes and pizzas, but during the refining process as much as 98 per cent of some key nutrients is lost. These foods provide calories, but have virtually no nutritional value – they have 'empty calories'.
- Liquid oils are processed into cheap, spreadable margarines and hydrogenated vegetable oils. The process (known as hydrogenation) completely alters the chemical structure of these fats, making it impossible for the body to recognize and process them. But, more worryingly, these 'killer' fats can have very serious health consequences[4], which include obesity, the build-up of LDL cholesterol and heart disease.
- Many fruits and vegetables – particularly those grown overseas, such as bananas and mangoes – are harvested before they've completed their growth cycle and ripened in an artificial environment, which depletes their nutrient content.
- Milk matters! In some countries, dairy herds are injected with oestrogenic hormones so that each cow can produce 98 or so pints (56 litres) of milk a day, rather than the 16 pints (9 litres) that nature intended. With the risk of breast cancer increasing year on year, we need to avoid excess oestrogen.

- Preservatives and pesticides are added to make our foods look more attractive and last longer.

Is it any wonder that degenerative disease levels are higher now than ever before?

The caveman diet – clues to the foods that may suit us best

We are descended from Palaeolithic man, who lived about 100,000 years ago. Studying his diet can provide real clues about the foods that may suit us best. He would not have had any fizzy drinks, fast food or pre-packaged food to pop into the microwave. He hadn't even heard of bread or potatoes.

Countless studies reveal that Palaeolithic man would have eaten a diet high in fruits and fibre-rich vegetables and seeds and, when the hunting was good,[5] he would have enjoyed plenty of lean meat[6]. The high fruit and vegetable content would have provided a rich source of vitamins and minerals. It was recently estimated that the typical diet of neo-Palaeolithic man supplied up to five times today's average intake of most vitamins and minerals. And in some cases – for example, vitamin A – his intake could be as high as 20 times today's average. He is likely to have eaten around 200 different varieties of fruit and vegetables. Today we seem to limit ourselves to around 15 common ones, such as broccoli, carrots and peas. Fats for the hunter-gatherer would have come from meat, seeds and occasionally fish. Fossil records indicate that rarely, if ever, did our human ancestors eat cereal grains or potatoes. It was not until around 10,000 years ago, with the development of agriculture, that diets high in carbohydrate grains, starches and dairy products became

common. That may seem like a long time, but in evolutionary terms it's the blink of an eye. Geneticists and evolutionary historians argue that our bodies have simply not yet had time to adjust to the increase in grains and dairy products that the agricultural revolution brought. This is one of the reasons why we can be quite intolerant to them.

Fertilizers are a legacy of war

Our diet has changed immeasurably from the hunter-gatherer foods we evolved to eat. The process has speeded up considerably since the end of the Second World War, when health requirements became of secondary importance to profit and growth, and farming methods took a disastrous turn for the worse. Only now is the price of all this becoming evident as we discover the effect of these fertilizers, pesticides and antibiotics which now dominate our foods.

The large industrial companies that supplied chemicals such as nitrates and phosphates for the munitions industry were left with huge stockpiles of these chemicals. Research had shown them that many plants seemingly grow well on a mixture of just three minerals: nitrogen (N), phosphorus (P) and potassium (K). And so began the growth of NPK fertilizers, which were by comparison much cheaper than traditional farming and soil-enhancement methods. By the 1960s organic farming had become hugely uneconomical and almost obsolete.

In the pre-war days, standard farming practices used manuring, mulching and crop rotation (i.e., organic) to ensure the soils were nutrient rich. These are the methods that have been around for thousands of years since agriculture began.

Unfortunately, although these fertilized crops will grow healthy and fine-looking produce, they are deficient in the other essential minerals such as selenium, chromium, magnesium, calcium, iron, iodine, zinc, cobalt, etc. Fertilizers are born of war and destruction, they are not conducive to health and vitality as they are lacking the vital minerals that are essential for human growth and nutrition. Also, these essential minerals become leached from the soil, which then becomes barren and devoid of goodness. Don't take my word for it, read Michael Colgan's *The New Nutrition*.

Primitive food combining?

Palaeolithic man's meals would not have looked the way ours do today. It seems unlikely that after wrestling with an antelope that he would have sloped off to find some tasty rice or roots to eat with his fare. He probably survived for days on meat alone and, while a supply of fresh meat was available, vegetables would have provided little attraction. After all, it might have been weeks before another successful hunt.

As far as the body is concerned, it is good to eat concentrated protein, like meat, in isolation from sugary and starchy carbohydrates, such as fruit, rice and root vegetables. Protein is primarily digested in the stomach, while starchy carbohydrate digests in the intestine. Protein and carbohydrates are each broken down by different enzymes that require different chemical conditions in order to function. The presence of protein slows down carbohydrate digestion, and vice versa. This has led some scientists and nutritionists to promote the food-combining ideology first devised by Dr Hay in the 1930s. Hay's theory was based upon the principle that

concentrated proteins like meat, eggs and dairy products should be eaten separately from starchy vegetable matter such as bread, potatoes and fruit. Our digestive systems do seem to function better when we eat this way. If you suffer from flatulence or bloating after a heavy meal, it's a good idea to think about adopting a food-combining approach.

Carb overload

Carbohydrate is the body's preferred source of fuel. Bread, pasta, rice, sugar, honey, fruit and vegetables are all sources of carbohydrate. The body breaks each down into glucose and, with the help of the hormone insulin, this is used for energy by the cells of the body. Quick-releasing or simple carbohydrates, such as pure sugar, sweets, honey and refined foods, like white bread and sugary cereals, may give you a short-term energy boost but they can also leave you feeling tired and irritable. When we overload on quick-releasing carbohydrate foods, we can suffer from weight gain, sugar cravings, stimulant craving and, ultimately, diabetes and obesity.

Sugar poisoning

Remember when Mummy warned you about the Honey Monster? Sugar is carbohydrate in its deadliest form. We are born with a sweet tooth, which should naturally be satisfied by wholesome, energy-rich foods like fruit. But cunning manufacturers have capitalized on our natural sweet tooth, and learned to extract the sweetness from these foods while leaving all the nutrients and fibre behind. Not only does refined sugar contain absolutely no nutrients, but it also utilizes the body's existing store of vitamins and minerals for its metabolism. This results in deficiencies and imbalances.[7, 8]

Sugar is the number-one additive used in the food industry. It is added to convenience foods, snacks, drinks and confectionery. On average we each consume around 135 lbs (61 kilos) of sugar every year – around 0.37 lbs (0.17 kilos) a day – when as little as two teaspoons in a day can have a detrimental effect on our blood chemistry. But we don't even realize how much sugar we are eating. Most of it is hidden in convenience foods! Check the ingredients on the back of that ready-made dinner you're just about to microwave or that fruit yoghurt and you might just be surprised to discover that sugar is high on the list. And it will not just be in the puddings! Remember that a teaspoon of sugar is equivalent to about 5 g. You will be amazed how much sugar is in the foods you regularly buy. It's everywhere!

Many scientific studies have revealed that a high-sugar diet contributes to kidney stones, arthritis, hardening of the arteries, cardiovascular disease, cataracts, headaches, fatigue, acne, premature ageing, behavioural changes (especially in children)[9] and a weakened immune system.

High levels of sugar in the circulating bloodstream disturb the body's physiology, and damage important structural proteins in the body. We normally have just a fraction of an ounce (3 g) of glucose circulating in our bloodstream. Our body is designed to cope with small fluctuations in glucose levels as we eat a meal containing meat and complex carbohydrates, which slowly release glucose into the bloodstream. So imagine how difficult it is for the body to cope with a sugar burst from a bar of chocolate. A recent study showed that 4 oz (110 g) of sugar (roughly the sugar content of a large bag of sweets) could suppress the immune system by as much as 50 per cent.[10] The *American Journal of Clinical Nutrition* reported that this effect occurred within five minutes, and lasted up to five hours.

Even an eternal optimist would struggle to find a good word to say about sugar. There is no positive benefit derived from the level of refined sugar in our diet. It should be omitted completely from your diet, or cut right back.

Hidden sugars
Carton of juice drink – 11 teaspoons of sugar
Can of coke – 9.8 teaspoons of sugar
Fruit yoghurt – 7.4 teaspoons of sugar
Sponge cake – 10.7 teaspoons of sugar

Sugar by another name
Most pre-packaged foods, from sauces to chicken in breadcrumbs to soft drinks, have some added sugar. It may be listed as:

Barley malt	Fructose
Cane sugar	Grape sugar
Concentrated fruit juice	Hydrolysed starch
Corn fructose	Maltose
Corn sweetener	Manitol
Corn syrup	Maple syrup
Demerara sugar	Polydextrose
Dextrin	Sucrose
Dextrose	

These are all types of sugar, and manufacturers often use these names on the food labels to disguise the amount of sugar in their products.

Syndrome X – The disease of the new millennium

Do you crave sugar and bread? Feel sluggish after eating? Find it impossible to lose weight? Feel irritable or dizzy without food? Lack energy? Has your doctor told you that you have high cholesterol or high blood pressure? If so, you may be suffering from an increasingly common collection of symptoms.

Scientists in reputed journals, such as the *American Journal of Clinical Nutrition*, *European Journal of Clinical Nutrition* and *The Lancet*, are now reporting on this cluster of symptoms, collectively referred to as Syndrome X. They can also be referred to as metabolic syndrome or Insulin Resistance Syndrome – IRS. The condition develops largely as a result of the body's inability to cope with both today's diet, which is too high in refined flour and sugar, and our sedentary, stressful lifestyle. Most people are still quite unaware of Syndrome X, but it affects most of us over the age of 30 to some degree. It is becoming increasingly common among clients at Bodydoctor Fitness.

The collection of Syndrome X symptoms include high blood pressure, high blood triglycerides (fats), high cholesterol, obesity and blood sugar disorders. Ultimately, these symptoms increase the likelihood of heart disease, Type II diabetes and even some cancers.

Insulin resistance

When we eat carbohydrates, whether in the form of fruits, vegetables or sweets, the body breaks down the carbohydrate into glucose, the body's main source of fuel. Insulin is the hormone produced by the pancreas to help the body absorb glucose from the bloodstream into the cells. When levels of insulin remain elevated for prolonged periods, as they will with a high-sugar, high-carbohydrate diet, the cells in the body become insensitive to the insulin, so glucose cannot be burned by the body for energy. This is known as insulin resistance, which is a prime factor in the development of Syndrome X. The body is forced to compensate by producing more and more insulin. Insulin doesn't just control blood sugar levels, it also controls appetite, fluid balance and growth hormone levels (which keep the body lean) and regulates the synthesis of cholesterol by the liver. So raised levels of insulin on a long-term basis have a number of serious physiological consequences. The control of fat metabolism, for example, can be disturbed, which leads to increased body fat and a heightened risk of heart disease. It also becomes increasingly difficult for the body to handle glucose and carbohydrate, which can result in symptoms of diabetes and higher blood pressure. Full-blown Syndrome X is then fast approaching – the Honey Monster's revenge!

Do you have any signs or symptoms of insulin resistance?

- Cravings for carbohydrates, sweets, fizzy drinks or stimulants like caffeine?
- History of yo-yo dieting and an inability to manage your weight; weight gain, particularly around the middle?
- Frequent urination and thirst?
- Disordered blood lipids – high cholesterol (above 240 mg/dl) or triglycerides (above 160 mg/dl)?
- A family history of diabetes?
- Symptoms of blood sugar imbalance (irritability, dizziness without food, cravings, difficulty waking, and drowsiness during the day)?

If you answered 'yes' to half of these questions, it is critically important that you avoid all sugar and limit quick-releasing carbohydrates in your diet (see 'What makes a healthy diet?' on page 204). Limit potatoes, bread and other starchy foods, and increase complex carbohydrate in the form of vegetables. You should also eat more protein from low-fat sources, such as chicken, pulses, yoghurt, cottage cheese and tofu.

The myth of the well-balanced diet

Countless studies have shown that we do not get enough micronutrients, such as vitamins, minerals and phytochemicals, from our diets. We need approximately 40 micronutrients to function at our best. In the UK we are, on average, deficient in a staggering six out of 10 key nutrients.[11]

Our basic requirements are currently measured against the recommended daily allowance, known as RDA. Using the RDA, research at the University of California estimates that half the American population is deficient in at least one of these nutrients and 20 per cent are deficient in all of them.

Recent government surveys in the UK showed that 89 per cent of children are not receiving the RDA for zinc; 47 per cent of women do not receive the RDA for folic acid and 72 per cent do not receive enough magnesium.[12] This situation is worse than it may at first appear. The term RDA is actually the amount of a nutrient necessary to avoid a deficiency disease. In some cases it is nothing like the amount we need for optimal health. The RDA for vitamin C, for example, is 60 mg. But research shows that between 1000–3000 mg a day would be required to help protect against

heart disease. That's up to 54 oranges a day (if they were organic and fresh!)

The nutrient content of our food is much lower than it used to be. Extensive farming has depleted the soil of minerals. But this is only the start of the problem. Fruits and vegetables, for example, are picked before they are ripe in order to allow time to be transported. Immediately they are doomed to contain a lower nutrient content than those allowed to ripen naturally on the tree or in the ground. Exposure to light and oxygen further reduces the nutrient content of fruit and vegetables, so that much of the vitamin content has been lost by the time they reach the supermarket shelves. Any additional processing further reduces vitamin levels. Pre-chopped carrots, for example, will have lost much of the vitamin content of the whole vegetable.

We need more!

Unfortunately, just as the nutrient content of our food has declined, the stresses of modern life mean that our daily requirement has increased dramatically. Everybody is affected: stressed business people need higher intakes of vitamin C and B5; children in built-up areas who are exposed to petrol fumes need more zinc and calcium than their cousins in the country; young women on the pill have an increased requirement for zinc, magnesium and vitamin B6; and smokers need all the anti-oxidant nutrients, especially vitamin C (a study published in 1991 showed that a smoker needs to consume four times the level of vitamin C than a non-smoker just to ensure they both have the same levels in their bloodstreams).[13] Exposure to an increased level of toxins, chemicals and pesticides also increases nutrient requirements as the liver struggles to detoxify.

Should we take supplements?

The answer is a definite 'yes'. Our bodies have a built-in defence system, but it only works properly if it receives the right levels of micronutrients. If it doesn't, then the body becomes vulnerable to a whole range of degenerative diseases. We find that we can't cope with stress, our get-up-and-go just gets up and disappears, and our moods swing. Our appearance suffers. We pile on the pounds, our hair looks lifeless and our nails start to chip. Now some doctors may argue that our bodies can get everything they need from a balanced diet, but this just isn't borne out by scientific research. Most people need a supplement of some sort. Of course, everybody is unique so ideally it's best to consult a nutritionist to discuss individual cases. But if this isn't possible, the best advice (supported in a recent edition of *Journal of the American Medical Association*) is that all adults should take a daily multivitamin. [14]

Getting back to basics

If what you've read so far isn't enough to make you cut out the junk and eat in a way that reflects your body's true design, I don't know what is! Perhaps the promise of increased energy, a sharper brain and a slimmer body? If you follow the simple suggestions in the following pages then I promise you all these benefits. Trust me! I'm the Bodydoctor!

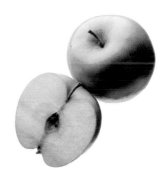

WHAT MAKES A HEALTHY DIET?

A FEW HANDY TIPS FOR A TIGHT BUM AND A FLAT TUM!

1)   Eat complex carbohydrates for energy.

2)   Eat enough protein.

3)   Increase the good fats and cut out the bad ones.

4)   Eat more alkaline-forming foods.

5)   Eat foods that are just the way nature intended them to be.

6)   Drink more water.

7)   Increase your vitamin and mineral intake.

Okay, so let's take each of these tips in turn ...

1 Complex carbohydrates for energy: eat your greens like Mum told you to

Choose whole grains, fresh fruits and vegetables and cut back (or out) refined white flour products such as pizza, pasta, white bread, cakes and biscuits.

Why is this important?

Carbohydrate is the body's preferred energy source. The body breaks all carbohydrates down into glucose, which it then uses as fuel to run itself. What it doesn't need for fuel is either stored as glycogen in the muscles and liver or gets converted into fat!

Carbohydrate comes in two forms. It can be simple or complex. Simple carbohydrates, which contain one or two sugar molecules, include refined sugar, some sweet vegetables, fruit and lactose (the sugar in milk). These are broken down rapidly by the body and give a quick burst of energy. Simple carbohydrates are also described as high-glycaemic carbohydrates because they release glucose into the blood quickly.

Complex carbohydrates, which contain long chains of molecules, include pulses, legumes, whole grains, green vegetables and some fruits. In fact, they probably include all the foods that our mothers forced us to eat when we were children because they were good for us. Admit it – they were right! These foods are classed as low-glycaemic index foods. They are good for our general vitality because they release glucose more slowly, give us more sustained energy and avoid rapid increases in blood sugar which, as I've already explained, can adversely affect long-term health.

Dump the junk

White bread, pasta, biscuits and the sugar that we add to tea and coffee are known as refined carbohydrates. They're called refined, because all the fibre that would normally slow down the release of sugar into the bloodstream has been stripped out. They behave as high-glycaemic index foods, and they have a dramatic effect on blood glucose levels. They may give you a quick energy burst, but ultimately you will end up feeling tired and craving sugar or stimulants, such as tea or coffee. They're no good – so cut them out of your diet now.

The insulin curve

The hormone insulin is produced when carbohydrates are digested. Insulin's basic function is to transport glucose from the blood into the cells. And it stands to reason that the more carbohydrates you eat, the more insulin the body produces. Unfortunately these high insulin levels prevent the body burning fat, and it will start to gain weight. The body also becomes confused with too much insulin circulating through the bloodstream, and may even over-produce insulin. This will push blood sugar levels too low (hypoglycaemia) and the body will then crave coffee, biscuits or sweet things to raise it again. Your body may eventually become resistant to insulin, and will need to produce more and more to get the desired effect and ultimately may become unable to manage glucose levels at all. This is when Type II diabetes becomes a real risk. Most current research blames high insulin levels for the sharp increase in obesity, heart disease and diabetes and the rise of Syndrome X. A low-glycaemic index diet will help avoid the long-term health risks associated with high insulin levels, and produce the optimal amount of fuel for the body.

Good Carbohydrate	Carbohydrate to limit	Carbohydrate to avoid
Green vegetables, peppers, tomatoes, onions and garlic Brown and basmati rice Quinoa Oats, rye and millet Pulses Cherries, apples, pears, grapefruit, plums, oranges and dried apricots	High-glycaemic index fruits and vegetables – pineapples, bananas, parsnips, potatoes, carrots and sweetcorn Starchy carbohydrates, such as potatoes, cereals and breads Fruit Juices Honey	Sugar and products containing it, including fizzy drinks, cakes and biscuits Wheat and wheat products like pasta and bread Processed breakfast cereals Refined wheat and grain products including white bread, biscuits and pasta

The low-glycaemic index diet (don't worry, it's not as bad as it sounds!)

- Avoid all refined carbohydrates and sugars. Cut out white bread, biscuits, cakes and fizzy drinks.
- Limit 'heavy' starchy carbohydrates, such as bread, pasta, potatoes and rice, to those meals you have just before exercising. The Bodydoctor Fitness Programme will soon burn off that excess glucose.
- Increase your intake of low-glycaemic index fruits and vegetables. Eat more green vegetables, bean sprouts, cucumber, lettuce, rocket, rhubarb, apples, pears, grapefruit, cherries and tomatoes.

See! It's not as hard as it sounds.

2 Get enough protein: meat and fish are the ideal dish

Increase sources of protein that are low in saturated fat such as fish, chicken, turkey, game meats, quinoa, tofu, nuts and seeds.

Protein is the building block of our bodies. Muscle is made of protein, which we need in order to develop and grow. That is also why it is important to eat some protein shortly after finishing a workout with the Bodydoctor Fitness Programme. It will help build muscle and repair the breakdown of tissues.

Protein is made up of amino acids, which are used to develop structural tissues, such as muscles, bones, ligaments, tendons, nails, hair and organs. Amino acids also feed the enzymes, hormones and neurotransmitters that control the body's basic physiology, immunity and mood.

There are 10 essential amino acids in protein. The body is unable to synthesize these naturally, and so the only way it gets them is through food. The following foods contain all 10 essential amino acids but have the added bonus that they are low in fat: eggs, beans, chicken, fish and lentils. There are also more exotic foods like quinoa, which is found in health shops and is similar to couscous, and soya. Game meats, such as pheasant, guinea fowl and venison, tend also to be lower in saturated fat than farmed animals.

Remember that old nursery rhyme about curds and whey that we learned as children? I didn't have a clue what it was then either, but I do now and it is one of the most valuable sources of protein – an absolutely amazing food supplement. Whey is produced as a by-product when cheese is manufactured. It is a particularly high-protein but low-fat source of essential amino acids. Researchers in Australia have found that the natural growth factors contained in whey protein can speed up the healing of bones, skin and muscle tissues.[15] It has also been clinically demonstrated to increase immunity,[16] help heal cataracts, improve cancer recovery and aid in the treatment of HIV. Whey protein powder is available at your local health food store. I usually recommend Whey to Go from Solgar (see Resources, page 260) which comes in several tasty flavours. Have a tub as a standby if you haven't eaten enough protein foods.

3 Increase the good fats and cut out the bad: eat the right fats for a trim body

Avoid saturated fats in snacks, fried food, dairy products and meat. Increase essential omega-3 and omega-6 oils found in oily fish and nuts and seeds and their oils.

Despite what some litigious Americans might claim, everybody knows that excess fat in the diet is a bad thing. If you eat too many fast-food meals then you will get fat but you may also become ill. Too much fat in the diet is one of the main factors blamed for the rise in heart disease, strokes and cancer in the Western world. But what most people don't realize is that some fats are actually good for you. In fact, they are essential. They can help the body

fight infection, improve your brain function, keep hormones in balance and maintain the health of cell membranes. Surprisingly these good fats may also help to keep your heart healthy.

If you suffer from any of the following, you probably don't have enough essential fats in your diet. It's time to increase your intake!

1) Dry or cracked skin (particularly on the heels); eczema; or you find that wounds take a long time to heal
2) Dull or brittle hair, or hair loss
3) Soft or brittle nails
4) Depression, irritability or mood swings, dyslexia or dyspraxia
5) Pre-menstrual syndrome, breast tenderness
6) Arthritis, aching joints or fatigue
7) Frequent infections or allergies
8) Difficulty losing weight, fatigue or lack of energy

Which are the good fats?

The good fats are polyunsaturated fats and monounsaturated fats.

The key polyunsaturated fats are the omega-3 and omega-6 essential fats, which are vital to maintaining general health. They boost the immune system, stimulate the metabolism, keep hormones in balance and the joints supple. These essential fats also keep the heart healthy and, as if that wasn't enough, keep our brains functioning and our moods in check. But the body cannot make these fats and so we need to eat the right foods to provide them. Omega-6 oils, which are found in nuts and seeds, evening primrose, starflower and borage oil, have been shown to prevent blood clots and keep the blood thin. They can also reduce inflammation and pain in the joints, and so are vital in preventing arthritis. Omega-3 oils, which are found in fish oils, linseed (flaxseed) oil, pumpkin seeds and walnuts, are particularly helpful in keeping the heart healthy. They help lower blood pressure, reduce blood stickiness and reduce cholesterol levels. Some people find that inflammatory conditions, such as arthritis and eczema, improve when they regularly have omega-3 oils. A simple tip? The best sources of these vital molecules are oily fish, such as tuna, mackerel, salmon and sardines.

Monounsaturated fats (also known as omega-9 fats) are also good fats. They are not deemed essential. Yet they can have health benefits. Olive oil is probably the best-known example of monounsaturated fat. It has been shown to lower bad cholesterol (also known as LDH) in the body, while raising the good cholesterol (HDL). Everybody always talks about the healthy Mediterranean diet. Well, olive oil is one of the main factors contributing to the low rate of heart disease in that region.

Which are the bad fats?

Saturated and hydrogenated fats are the ones to avoid. Now that won't be easy – fast foods, ready-made cakes, biscuits and packaged dinners are packed with saturated fats and hydrogenated oils and they frequently lack any essential fatty acids. Saturated fats are also found in all animal products (which makes it difficult to cut them out completely) and many vegetable oils. Many margarine brands contain hydrogenated fats.

Saturated fats can raise the level of cholesterol in your blood and contribute to heart disease and cancer. They also slow down the liver's ability to remove the artery-clogging LDL (or bad) cholesterol. A diet high in saturated fat can

also stimulate oestrogen over-production, leading to female pre-menstrual and hormonal problems.

Food manufacturers like to harden oils to make them solid at room temperature, thereby extending their shelf life. They do this by a process known as hydrogenation. When oils are hydrogenated the chemical structure is altered, which makes them difficult for the body to assimilate. Hydrogenated fats can also disrupt the body's ability to use vital essential fatty acids. For this reason, avoid them completely. Using butter (in moderation), however, may actually be preferable to some margarines, because many of them contain hydrogenated fat. Check your usual brand – if the ingredients list includes hydrogenated fats, throw it out.

Five ways to get enough good fats

1) Eat oily fish, such as tuna, mackerel, salmon, herring, sardines or sild (young herring), two or three times a week
2) Eat a tablespoon of mixed seeds (or their cold pressed oils) every day: pumpkin, sunflower, sesame, hemp or linseed (flax)
3) Avoid hydrogenated oils in margarines and processed foods
4) Reduce or avoid saturated fat where possible
5) Take an essential fatty acid supplement, which contains all the essential oils (try Udo's Choice, or Higher Nature Essential Balance (see Resources, page 260)

4 Keep your body alkaline!

Eat more alkaline-forming foods, such as fruit, vegetables, sprouted seeds and certain nuts, and cut back on acid-forming foods, such as meat, fish, eggs, grains and cheese.

The body functions best when it is in an

alkaline state. But just to make things difficult, our metabolism actually produces acid. In order to achieve the health and vitality we all want, it is important to counteract this acidity with alkaline foods.

A residual 'ash' is left when the body breaks down food. The elements found in this ash will determine whether the food has an acid- or alkaline-forming effect on the body. Foods like eggs, grains, cheese and concentrated protein (such as meat and fish) leave acidic ash in the body, while stress, smoking and drinking alcohol also create acid. It is vital that you eat more alkaline-forming foods, such as fruit and vegetables, to counteract this. A grilled steak, for example, should be eaten with lots of vegetables to balance out the acid that it creates in the body.

Four ways to keep your body alkaline

1) Increase your intake of fruit, vegetables and less-concentrated protein foods, like beans, seeds, lentils and legumes
2) Cut back on concentrated proteins, such as cheese, eggs, meat and fish, and gluten grains, like wheat and rye
3) Cut back on smoking and drinking

5 Can't read, don't need!

Look at the lists of ingredients on the packet or tin. If you can't read it, the chances are that your body can't process it!

Eating foods that come naturally

Eat foods that are just the way nature intended. It stands to reason that something that is completely natural is likely to be better for you than something that has been manufactured, such as processed meats and vegetables, and

pre-packaged ready meals and snacks. Choose a cut of organic pork over a sausage, or a crispy lettuce over the prepared, ready-washed variety. Go for a cup of herbal tea rather than a glass of lemonade.

As I've already pointed out, most prepared meals contain high levels of sugar and saturated fats. They are also likely to contain preservatives, additives and hydrogenated oils, which the body is unable to process and which blocks its ability to make use of healthy polyunsaturated oils.

* Buy fruit and vegetables that come loose, not pre-packaged.
* Choose seasonal fruit and vegetables
* Opt for organic foods. They may be more expensive, but they are free from preservatives and additives.
* Try to eat half your (loose and seasonal) fruit and vegetables raw. Raw food is full of vital vitamins, minerals and enzymes to aid digestion.
* Buy British. Imported food may have been harvested before it was ripe and will have lost nutrients during transport. An orange can lose up to 80 per cent of its vitamin C content by the time it reaches the supermarket shelves.
* Avoid ready meals and processed foods. I know I'm being repetitive here, but my job is to tell you what you need to know – not what you want to hear.

6 Drink more water

Drink at least eight glasses of pure water a day. Water makes up 70 per cent of the body. All physiological processes, including digestion, circulation and excretion, are influenced by the level of water in our bodies. Unfortunately it is not always easy to tell whether the body is properly hydrated. 'Ah!' I hear you say. 'I know when my body doesn't have enough water because I feel thirsty!' If only it were that easy. Research shows that we don't actually feel thirsty until the body is already in a state of quite advanced dehydration.[17] Mild dehydration can cause fatigue, headaches, dizziness and poor concentration. You should drink at least eight glasses of water every day just to keep the body hydrated – and that does not include teas (unless they are herbal) or coffees. Along with alcohol (which also does not count in the glasses tally), tea and coffee act as diuretics, which can promote water loss. You will know that you are drinking enough water if your urine is a pale colour. A word of warning, though: the vitamin B in some multi-vitamins can turn your urine bright yellow!

If you are undertaking the Bodydoctor Fitness Programme, you'll need to increase your intake of water. Recent research shows that dehydration reduces skeletal muscle endurance by 18 per cent,[18] so you will get more out of your training sessions if you make sure that you are drinking enough. Always take a bottle of water to the gym! A good rule of thumb is to drink an extra half litre for every half-hour that you exercise.

7 Get your vitamins and minerals

Vitamins and minerals are classed as micronutrients, because they are needed in tiny amounts. They act as co-factors, helping all the chemical reactions in the body to occur. Vitamins and minerals work in partnership, so a single deficiency can affect your mood, energy levels, hormone balance or even your resistance to infection. Read on to find out how.

Vitamins from A to Z

Vitamins A, C and E are antioxidants, helping to protect the body's cells from damage by radiation, chemical reactions in the body, infections, cancer and even ageing. If your body doesn't get enough antioxidant nutrients then you may become vulnerable to recurrent infections, premature ageing, heart disease or even cancer. Specifically, vitamin E guards circulating cholesterol against the oxidation effects that contribute towards heart disease.

The B-vitamin family aids the release of energy from food and helps balance the levels of the brain's neurotransmitters – the chemicals that allow the brain's cells to talk to each other. So it's not surprising that they also control your mood and state of mind. People suffering from depression or anxiety are often deficient in B vitamins.

Zinc is involved in just about every bodily function you can think of. Zinc can help balance hormones, aid digestion, help growth, control moods and boost immunity levels, yet many people are zinc-deficient. White marks on the fingernails are the most common symptom, but did you realize that stretch marks can also be a sign of zinc deficiency? And if you lack appetite or suffer from depression or emotional problems, allergies, acne or even infertility, then it's likely that you're not getting enough zinc in your diet.

Magnesium, which is found in leafy green vegetables, is important for healthy bones, hormone balance and production, and controlling muscular contractions. But 72 per cent of women and 42 per cent of men do not get enough of it. Deficiency signs include pre-menstrual symptoms, constipation, lack of energy or even muscle tremors.

The trouble is that, while you may now realize you are deficient in certain micronutrients, it is hard to know what is the right level for your body. Your own biochemistry and lifestyle will dictate whether you need more or less of a particular vitamin or mineral. One way to accurately assess your needs is to visit a nutritionist, who will take a detailed health history and examine your lifestyle. He or she may even carry out a sweat or hair mineral analysis to assess your nutrient status. Alternatively, increasing your intake of all fruits and vegetables, especially green leafy ones like lettuce, kale, cabbage and lettuce, will help. You can also take a multivitamin and mineral as insurance.

Lose the lard and lighten up

It's official: we're getting fatter! A recent report from the Medical Research Council's Centre for Nutrition revealed that 50 per cent of the adult population is overweight. One in five of us is clinically obese.[19] The British Nutrition Federation predicts that if current trends continue, over half the British population will be clinically obese by 2030.[20] At any one time, 45 per cent of women and 30 per cent of men are actively seeking to lose weight. But in most cases it isn't working.[21] They haven't been to The Bodydoctor yet!

Fad diets do not work

The truth is that most of us put back on weight within a year of losing it. And sometimes we put on more than we lost.

But let's dispel some of the myths about weight loss.

If you want to lose weight, avoid fat in your diet. FALSE!

As I've already explained (see page 207) our bodies do need some fats. They need the essential fats in oily fish and seeds but they do not need saturated fat. Dr Udo Erasmus, the brilliant author of *Fats That Heal, Fats That Kill,* discovered that eating more essential fats actually leads to an increased metabolic rate which allows the body to burn more calories. If your body is deprived of all fats then it will go into starvation mode. It will increase the production of lipoprotein lipase, which is an enzyme that collects and stores fat. The next time you eat fat, your body will go into overdrive and increase fat deposition to protect it against any future deprivations.

A low-calorie diet will make me lose weight. FALSE!

If you severely restrict calories you may get rapid weight loss, but your metabolic rate will slow down and you'll cannibalize lean muscle tissue. On a low-calorie diet, 45 per cent of weight loss can come from muscle.[22] Lean muscle burns fat. If you reduce lean muscle, your metabolic rate goes down and you burn fat more slowly. Because your metabolism has slowed down, when you eat normally you pile the weight back on – and more besides. Low-calorie diets also restrict nutrient intake, leading to nutrient deficiencies. None of us can starve ourselves. You will eventually reach for the biscuits and damn – you've blown your calorie intake for the day, so you might as well eat the lot! If you recognize this pattern you will know that dramatically restricting calories just isn't sustainable.

From the sandwich shop	Foods to take to work
Salads	Health food bars such as Trophy seed bars or Jordan's Organic Crunch bars – both are wheat-free and don't contain much sugar
Yoghurt	
Fresh Fruit	Fresh fruit – cherries, berries, apples, pears, oranges, bananas
Smoothies	Snack-size bags of seeds
If there is no alternative but to have bread, choose wholemeal with a protein filling such as chicken, houmous or egg	Nuts
	Natural Yoghurt
	Slices of cold chicken, rice or oatcakes and a pot of houmous or cottage cheese
	Crudités of carrot, baby corn, cucumber, pepper and broccoli spears with reduced-fat houmous or cottage cheese

Missing lunch helps me lose weight. FALSE!

You need to eat regularly to maintain your blood sugar levels. If you miss meals then you will get tired and shaky as your blood sugar falls. This makes it very difficult to avoid being tempted by that stodgy muffin at 4 o'clock. Enjoying three smaller, healthier meals a day and the occasional healthy snack is a much better alternative to cutting out lunch.

Drinking strong coffee stops me feeling hungry and helps me lose weight. FALSE!

Drinking coffee disrupts blood sugar balance. Blood sugar highs and lows lead to tiredness and cravings for sugar and refined carbohydrates. If you are really serious about following the Bodydoctor Fitness Programme, cut out coffee. Full stop. No ifs. No buts. Just do it.

A high-protein, low-carbohydrate diet is the answer. FALSE!

There is a lot to be said for the insulin balancing effect of increasing protein and reducing carbohydrate. Generally, people have more energy and feel more alert when they do this. But I am against the gimmick versions of this diet – the ones that tell you to cut out fruit and vegetables and eat as much cream, cheese and fried red meat as you want. That clearly cannot be good for your health. And it can make your breath smell like a dead cat.

Are you suffering from blood sugar imbalance?

Blood sugar imbalance leads to tiredness, irritability and cravings. It is often the hidden reason for failing to stick to a healthy eating regime. Get your blood sugar to remain even throughout the day, and you'll find it much easier to burn fat and avoid succumbing to the sweet temptation of cakes and biscuits.

- Do you feel dizzy and irritable without food?
- Do you get cold sweats?
- Do you feel drowsy during the day?
- Are you addicted to sweet foods?
- Are you excessively thirsty?
- Do you need something to get you going in the morning?
- Do you have tea, coffee, foods and drinks that contain sugar, or cigarettes at regular intervals during the day?
- Do you sometimes lose concentration?
- Do you have less energy than you would like?

Two recent studies in the *New England Journal of Medicine* found that slimmers following high-protein, low-carbohydrate diets initially lost more weight than those on calorie-restricted, low-fat diets. But the studies also discovered a high drop-out rate and found that after one year the differences in weight loss were not that significant between the two diets.[23, 24]

Foods labelled 'low fat' will help me lose weight. FALSE!

I am sorry to say this to you, but 'low fat' processed foods are often packed with sugar and refined carbohydrates. If you eat more carbohydrate than you need, or if your insulin levels remain high (as they will if you eat a lot of sugar) then you will not lose weight.

Basically, our bodies need all the major food groups. Cutting out any one group will leave your body unbalanced, and is just not sustainable long-term. You need to eat enough calories to avoid your body going into starvation mode. Weight (fat) loss needs to be slow to allow your body to adjust gradually. You should not lose more than 2 lb (or 1 kg, if you prefer) a week.

Handy tips for permanent fat loss!

Cut out sugar and refined carbohydrates

After reading everything that I've already said about refined carbohydrates and sugars, I'm sure you've already dumped them from your diet! But just in case you are still in denial, here's a little reminder about why you should cut out all refined sugar and limit high-glycaemic index carbohydrates (see page 206). They cause rapid rises in insulin. Remember? When insulin levels are high your body is in fat-storage mode and just cannot burn fat; quite simply, you won't lose weight.

Increase fibre

Fibre from plant sources like fruit, vegetables and grains makes you feel fuller and slows down the release of glucose and fat from food. If you follow the Bodydoctor Nutrition Plan™ then you should get enough fibre. But you could also try konjac fibre, which is extracted from a tropical fruit. Although clinical trials have so far proved inconclusive, it does seem to control blood sugar fluctuations and make people feel fuller, so controlling appetite.

Get enough essential fatty acids. Avoid all saturated fats

Have a tablespoon of mixed seeds, such as pumpkin, sunflower, sesame or linseed, a day. Use bottled cold-pressed seed oil for salads. An ideal oil is Udo's Choice, which contains the right balance of omega-3 and omega-6 essential oils (see page 207).

Consider a helping hand from supplements

Unfortunately nothing can replace the hard work of exercise and diet – no matter what some of those 'magic pills' might claim. But, while those should be avoided at any cost, there are certain natural substances that you might consider adding to your diet to help metabolize fat. If you are taking any medication, always seek your doctor's advice before taking any supplements.

Chromium, a mineral found in whole grains and Brewers' yeast, works with insulin to stabilize blood sugar levels, which can help control weight and appetite. Our average daily intake is under 50 mcg, but the optimum level is around 200 mcg. Two studies carried out at Bemidgi State University in Minnesota showed that a daily 200 mcg dose of chromium not only helped burn fat but also, if used in combination with an exercise programme, helped to build muscle.[25]

If you suffer from any of the symptoms of blood sugar highs and lows or insulin resistance you should definitely consider the help of extra chromium. But a word of warning! Since the 2003 Food Standards Association report on the safety of vitamins and minerals, the chromium polynicotinate form is generally considered safer than chromium picolinate.

L-carnitine is an amino acid found in muscle tissue. It transports fat to the mitochondria (the powerhouses of the cell) where it is burned. The amount of fat burned depends on the level of L-carnitine in the muscle. But it can get rapidly depleted by exercise, so an L-carnitine supplement will help!

A study published in 1985 showed that some athletes significantly increased their use of fat during exercise when supplementing their diets with 2 g per day of L-carnitine.[26]

Hydroxy Citrate (HCA) is extracted from the rind of the tamarind fruit and has been used for centuries as a spice in Asia. But it also inhibits the enzyme that converts sugar into fat stores. In fact, evidence suggests HCA can cut the conversion of excess carbohydrate to fat by 70 per cent over 8–12 hours.

Participants in one eight-week trial showed 5 lb (2.3 kg) more weight loss on average than individuals in a control group taking dummy pills.[27] Because HCA reduces fat production, it may be useful for individuals wanting to control cholesterol and blood triglyceride (fat) levels.

CLA is a type of polyunsaturated fat found in dairy foods, meat and sunflower seeds. It helps the body to burn fat and build lean muscle. CLA increases the activities of enzymes that encourage the release of fat from storage in order to allow it to be burned as fuel. While weight-loss trials have been inconclusive, CLA has still been shown to help build lean body mass.

The best sources of CLA are dairy products and lamb. However, because these are also high in saturated fat, it is better to take CLA as a supplement.

For your own prescription of the above supplements, visit our website: www.bodydoctor.com

THE BODYDOCTOR NUTRITION PLAN™

SOME SIMPLE PRINCIPLES

Incorporate these changes gradually, over a 10-day period. If you try to change your life in a day, you'll want your old life back in a week!

- Do not weigh yourself

- Stop counting calories

- Focus on eating the foods that your body is designed to eat

- Cut out foods such as sugar and refined carbohydrates

- Eat more fruits, vegetables and new grains (e.g., quinoa and rye)

- Be relaxed about the changes you are making to your diet

- Don't panic if you have an occasional lapse! You're only human!

The Bodydoctor says:

'Follow these principles as closely as possible during the six-week intensive exercise programme. Then make these new habits a part of your life every day. You will feel great — trust me!'

THE GOLDEN RULES

All you need is on this page and the reverse. Cut it out of the book or photocopy it. Have it encapsulated. Put it where you can see it – on the fridge or the inside of the kitchen cupboard. Follow the rules.

1. Don't skip meals.
Eat three main meals a day and two healthy snacks. This maintains your blood sugar levels, avoiding the highs and lows that leave you feeling tired and will have you reaching for the first chocolate biscuit you can find!

2. Always include low-fat protein in your breakfast
Start the day with a good breakfast. Including low-fat protein, such as yoghurt, cottage cheese, egg or seeds (see the recipes on page 228), will help balance both your blood sugar levels and moods. You'll keep going for longer. You must also include complex carbohydrates before you work out.

3. Eat complex carbs before your workout, and protein afterwards
I've said this in my workout Golden Rules (see page 73), and I'll do so again: you need complex carbohydrates, such as porridge oats, wholegrain bread or rye bread for energy before you exercise, or you won't have enough immediate energy reserves to draw upon. Always eat protein (or take a protein supplement, see page 206) within 1½–1¾ hours maximum after you've finished. You need protein to replenish lost muscle protein that's been depleted during your workout.

4. Cut out all sugar and refined carbohydrate, like biscuits, cakes, white bread and refined cereals

5. Try to fill at least half of your plate with vegetables
Vegetables, including some raw varieties, should form the bulk of your two main meals. Try to include as many different varieties over the week as you can (see the shopping lists on page 221).

6. Drink at least eight glasses (1½ litres) of water a day
Cut out diuretics such as tea and coffee, which encourage water loss. Herbal teas are fine. Why not experiment with the huge selection of herbal and fruit teas available in supermarkets and health food shops? I particularly like peppermint, lemon and ginger, blackcurrant and the range of yogi teas with liquorice (see Resources for suppliers, page 260).

7. Supplement your deficiencies
The very minimum you should take every day is a good multivitamin. (See Resources for recommended suppliers, page 260). If you are on any prescribed medication, consult your doctor before taking any supplements.

8. Eat your food in as natural a state as possible
How close to your natural optimum state would you feel if you'd been dumped into boiling water for half an hour? Eating fruits and vegetables as close to raw as possible preserves all the natural goodness – enzymes, vitamins and minerals – in your food. When it's overcooked, it's just pulp with little nutrient content. Similarly, choose to grill, steam or stir-fry when you cook to minimize the calories and maximize the nutrient content of what you are preparing.

Fuel for exercise: what to eat and when

The Bodydoctor Fitness Programme will intensify as you progress, so your energy levels will be higher but you'll also need more energy resources. To make the most of your training programme, you need to fuel your body correctly at the right times. People get better results when they include a source of complex carbohydrate, such as oats or sweet potato, in the meal before exercising. This provides the glucose that powers your muscles.

If you exercise in the morning, have oats or rye bread with your breakfast. If you prefer to work out later in the day, choose baked sweet potato, brown rice or pulses, for example, for your lunch or evening meal. It is essential to eat some protein, such as a tuna steak or stir-fried chicken, within 1½–1¾ hours maximum after exercising. If you can't make a meal, at least have a whey protein shake, such as Whey to Go from Solgar (see Resources, page 260). The protein works to repair and build new muscle fibres.

What should I be eating?

Water on waking

Drink a glass of hot water with lemon juice as soon as you wake. This stimulates the liver, clears out toxins and helps alkalize the system. Don't forget to eat breakfast every day, and take your supplements then. It is important not to take supplements on an empty stomach as this can make you feel quite sick.

Vegetables and fruit

Vegetables and fruit will form the majority of what you eat. They are alkaline-forming, full of fibre and packed with vitamins and minerals. Invest in a juicer! Freshly prepared juices are an ideal way to increase your fruit and vegetable intake.

If you are not sure which fruits and vegetables are better for you, just try to eat as big a range of colours as you can.

- Red, orange, yellow and purple ones, like peppers, berries and carrots, are packed full of immune-boosting phytochemicals, like the antioxidants lycopene and anthocyanidins, and bioflavonoids, which support the immune system.
- Green leafy vegetables, such as spinach, kale, watercress, rocket and lettuce, are a very rich source of magnesium and iron.
- Sprouted seeds, such as alfalfa or mung beans, are packed with vitamins, minerals and plant enzymes and have an alkalizing effect on the body.
- Onions and garlic are natural antibiotics – they're very cleansing, and can actually help lower cholesterol.
- Cruciferous vegetables, such as broccoli, cauliflower, kale and Brussels sprouts, are good sources of vitamins and assist hormone balance and detoxification.
- Citrus fruits, like grapefruits and oranges, are good sources of vitamin C, beta-carotene and bioflavonoids.
- Apples are a good source of vitamin C and pectin, which binds to toxic-heavy metals like mercury and lead and helps carry them out of the body. Pectin may also help lower cholesterol levels, and is proven to be good for arthritis, rheumatism and gout.

Lean meat and fish

Eat oily fish, such as salmon, mackerel, herring and tuna, which provide a good source of omega-3 essential fats. These fats are particularly important for boosting your brain power and protecting against cardiovascular disease.

It is always better to buy organic chicken or turkey because they avoid the excess hormones that non-organic poultry are commonly exposed to. It also tastes nicer.

Game, such as pheasant, guinea fowl and venison, is particularly healthy, as it tends to be lower in saturated fat than meat like pork, beef and lamb.

Complex carbohydrates

Complex carbohydrates, such as brown rice, whole grains (millet, rye, buckwheat and oats) and green vegetables are the best sources of energy as they are not rapidly digested and so release glucose slowly. This maintains energy levels and avoids blood sugar highs and lows, which I've already warned can prove detrimental to a healthy eating programme.

Vegetarian protein sources

Don't forget vegetarian sources of protein, such as quinoa, tofu, brown rice, beans, lentils, seeds, nuts and eggs. These are more easily digested and tend to be lower in fat than meat and dairy products.

If you are vegetarian, remember that you need to eat complete protein in order to get the full requirement of amino acids. In practice, this means eating some eggs or combining beans and pulses with corn, nuts, rice or seeds.

Water

I'll say it again – drink at least eight glasses (1½ litres) of water a day, and more if you are training (see page 79). If you increase your water intake you'll improve your concentration, energy levels, mental function and athletic performance.

Essential fats

Omega-6 and omega-3 essential fatty acids are vital for keeping us healthy (see page 207). Every day, you should include one of the following:

- An essential oil supplement (try to find one that includes a source of both omega-3 and omega-6 oils).
- One tablespoon of mixed seeds.
- A portion of oily fish, such as mackerel, salmon or tuna.
- A tablespoon of Essential Balance or Udo's Choice oil (see Resources, page 260) which should be added to salad or food. Beware, though! Do not try to cook with these oils as they are very unstable at high temperatures. Similarly, don't add them to very hot food.

Non-dairy milks and butter

Reduce or avoid milk and try out some of the non-dairy alternatives, such as oat, soya or rice milk. Trust me! You'll hardly taste the difference if you use these milks on cereals or in smoothies. Tahini, which is made from sesame seeds, is also a good substitute for butter.

Good snacks

- Ryvita with cottage cheese
- Bowl of cherries, blueberries or raspberries
- Natural yoghurt with apple or pear
- Almonds (about 10) with an apple, pear or berries
- Oat biscuit with tahini, houmous or avocado dip
- Mixed nuts and dried fruits, like apricots
- Rice cake with tahini, houmous or avocado dip.
- Rice cakes release glucose quickly so it is best to make sure you combine these with protein

Food fixes

Do you have:

A big tum?

What makes you swell and feel like hell?
If you suffer from any digestive complaints,
such as flatulence, bloating, constipation or
diarrhoea, or if you are having problems losing
weight try cutting out all refined sugars and
limiting the amount of wheat you eat. Then you
may find that separating dense proteins (like
cheese, egg, fish and meat) from starchy
carbohydrates (like rice, potatoes and bread)
helps. These dense proteins are hard to digest
and this is certainly the way our ancestors
would have consumed meat. Digestive enzymes
in supplement form may also help alleviate
flatulence and bloating.

Big tum, fat bum? No Fun!

What should you avoid in your diet?
The answer is refined carbohydrates.
Unfortunately, these are all the comfort foods,
like cakes, biscuits, sweets, fizzy drinks, jams
and spreads, white bread, pasta, pastry and pizza.
But refined carbohydrate causes a rapid rise in
blood sugar, which may give you a quick energy
burst, but over time will leave you feeling tired
and craving more sugar or stimulants, such as
coffee and tea, to keep you going.

Sugar! Cut out all the added sugar in your diet.
Eat fresh fruit if you want something sweet and
try Panda liquorice bars, natural fruit bars or
sesame-seed snacks for an occasional treat.

Stimulants! Avoid caffeine in coffee, cola,
stimulant drinks and tea. Caffeine triggers the
release of stimulatory neurotransmitters. In the

short term it will give you a boost, but long
term it can upset your blood sugar balance,
leaving you feeling tired and craving sugary,
refined foods. It becomes a vicious circle.

Wheat! Avoid wheat – we are not designed to
eat it. Most people feel better when they cut
out wheat from their diet. There are now lots of
delicious alternatives, such as rye bread, millet
cereals, quinoa (similar to couscous), buckwheat
pasta, oat and rice cakes.

Dairy! Cow's milk is produced by cows for
cows, not people. Many of us are unable to cope
with the protein in milk (known as casein) or
the sugar (lactose). This can lead to digestive
discomfort, constipation and excess mucus
which may just give you a permanent 'blocked
up' feeling, but can also lead to glue ear and
sinusitis.

Reduce or avoid all milk and cheese products
except for cottage cheese and yoghurt, which
are partially digested, making it easier for the
body to cope with. A live natural bio-yoghurt is
preferable as it contains a source of beneficial
gut flora.

Alcohol! Cut it out if at all possible. It's high
in calories, and also disturbs blood sugar
balance and sleep patterns. Experiment with
non-alcoholic alternatives, such as Aqua Libra
and Amé, but avoid low-alcohol beers as these
contain lots of chemicals that are not conducive
to good health.

Processed foods and preservatives!
IF YOU CAN'T READ IT, YOUR GUTS
DON'T NEED IT.
I know I'm going on about this, but start
reading the labels on everything you're
tempted to buy. If there are lots of ingredients
you don't understand, just put the packet
back on the supermarket shelf. Our diets
and environment are full of chemicals and
compounds that are toxic to the body. Eat
fewer processed and packaged foods
wherever possible.

Need to add, the food is bad
Just take a look at what this lot of poisonous
addictive junk can be held responsible for. Check
out the ingredients in some of your children's
favourite sweets and fast foods. That's the Honey
Monster laid bare for all to see.

E102–E133 – Azo-dyes:
Some of these have been shown to reduce
mineral levels, reduce digestive enzyme activity
and unbalance neurotransmitter balance, leading
to hyperactivity in children, irritability, sleep
disturbances and reduced attention span.

E310 – Aspartame:
Artificial sweetener found in products such as
Canderel, Nutrasweet, Toothkind, Diet Coke,
Pepsi-lite, low-cal squashes, juices and yoghurts.
Aspartame is an excitatory neurotransmitter.

Research into the effects of aspartame is
controversial. However, it is best avoided.

E621 – MSG:
Symptoms that have been ascribed to MSG include
behavioural problems in children, depression,
irritability, thirst, asthma, insomnia, skin rashes,
dizziness and fatigue.

E210–E219 – Benzoates:
Used as preservatives in a wide range of foods,
beverages and pharmaceuticals. Benzoal peroxide
is used primarily as a bleaching agent in the
manufacture of white flour, white bread, lecithin
(used as an emulsifier) and some cheeses.

Sulphites, nitrates and nitrites:
Used as preservatives. Best avoided because of
their long-term health effects.

SHOPPING JUST GOT GOOD FOR YOU

Shopping is your pit stop on the path to salvation. Here's what to buy. And if you're tempted to stray off the path, just remember: 'flat tum, firm bum, round bum, buy some!' You can photocopy this card. Have it encapsulated and take it with you when you shop. It works! There will always be something there to remind you.

Vegetables
Sweet potato
Celeriac
Spinach
Lettuce
Kale
Endive
Chicory
Mange tout
Red peppers
Avocado (limit to
    one a week)
Onions
Carrots
Garlic
Ginger
Celery
Beetroot
Asparagus
Bean sprouts
Broccoli
Cauliflower
Watercress
Spinach
Pumpkin
Brussels sprouts
Bok choy

Pulses
Lentils
Chickpeas
Flageolet beans
Butter beans
Chickpeas
Kidney beans
Black-eyed beans

Grains
Rye bread, e.g.,
    Borodinsky's
    rye bread and Terence
    Stamp wheat-free
    bread
Rice cakes
Oat cakes
Brown rice
Ryvita
Amaranth
Quinoa

Cereals
Millet flakes, e.g.,
    Mesa Sunrise
Porridge oats
Wheat-free muesli

Seeds and nuts
Sunflower

Sesame
Linseed
Pumpkin
Hemp
Almonds
Brazil nuts

Fruits
Cherries
Apples
Pears
Oranges
Tropical fruits
Bananas
Cantaloupe melon

Citrus fruits
Strawberries
Tomatoes
Blackberries
Apricots
Grapefruit
Kiwi fruit
Lemons
Limes
Peaches
Plums
Figs
Prunes

Meat
Organic chicken
Venison
Guinea fowl
Pheasant

Fish
All fish, but especially:
Tuna
Salmon
Prawns
Mackerel
Herring

Drinks
Bottled water — still and
    sparkling
Selection of herbal teas
Dandelion coffee
Rooibosch (Red bush
    tea)
Amé, Aqua Libra or
    Purdey's

Oils
Cold-pressed olive oil
Udo's Choice, Flax oil or
    hemp seed oil
Sesame seed oil

Foods to avoid	Alternatives
Sugar	Fresh fruit, dried apricots, liquorice and natural fruit bars
Wheat	Millet flakes, corn pasta, quinoa, buckwheat, oats, rye bread, rice bread and rice cakes
Milk and hard cheese	Rice milk, oat milk and soya milk products, yoghurt and cottage cheese
Foods high in saturated fats, such as sausages, red meat, crisps and snacks	Aim to grill food. Snack on nuts, seeds, fruit and popcorn
Coffee	Herbal teas, rooibosch tea, coffee substitutes and home-made juices

Eating plans

This section gives you the nutrition basics rather than a prescription diet: I've included detailed menus for two weeks and a collection of recipes so you can pick and choose as your taste and mood dictates. You don't need to follow the menus to the letter – simply use them as a source of ideas as you develop the Plan to suit your lifestyle. You can do it. You're on the road to a new you!

On waking

Start the day with a glass of hot water and lemon juice. This stimulates the liver and helps alkalize the system (see page 209). Ideally, drink your lemon water half an hour before eating breakfast.

Breakfast

You must eat breakfast every day, and it needs to include protein (see page 228). Protein helps regulate blood sugar balance, and it's also responsible for making the neurotransmitters in the brain that make us feel alert and motivated. Just adding a few seeds or nuts can make a difference to how you feel throughout the morning. If you tend to feel bloated or are slow to get going first thing, limit your breakfast bread and cereal.

Lunch

If you're prone to an afternoon slump, go easy on bread and pasta at lunchtime. Choose a large green salad with a small piece of fish or a few tablespoons of cottage cheese, and you will be amazed just how alert you feel after lunch. Try to fill at least half of your plate with salad, green vegetables or other low-glycaemic index vegetables (see page 206). Add a few tablespoons of chickpeas, flageolet beans or other pulses, as they give you steady energy release throughout the afternoon. If you're really organized in the morning, make up a lunch box with some of the following:

- Sandwich made from rye bread, and spread with tahini instead of butter
- Chicken satay sticks
- Vegetable crudités
- Brown rice and tuna salad
- Small piece of flapjack
- Dried apricots
- Melon slices, grapes, cherries or other convenient fresh fruit
- Cherry tomatoes
- Chicken drumstick or breast (without the skin if you are serious about losing weight!)

Evening meal

Don't eat a large meal late in the evening as the food will sit heavily in your stomach and you won't have any opportunity to use up the calories you've consumed. Choose a serving of protein-rich food, such as tofu, cottage cheese, meat, fish or prawns, and balance it with a similar-sized portion of carbohydrate food, such as brown rice, sweet potato, sweetcorn, corn on the cob, corn pasta, rye bread or heavy grain bread. Fill half of the plate with low-glycaemic index vegetables, such as broccoli, spinach, kale, lettuce, runner beans, courgette, garlic, tomatoes, mushrooms, peppers and mange tout.

Eating in restaurants

Your eating programme needs to be adaptable to suit your lifestyle. When you do find yourself in the Indian or Chinese, here are some hints!

Indian – Choose chicken tikka, dahl, chicken or prawn shashlick, raita, vegetable dishes, basmati rice. Avoid naan breads and creamy sauces.

Italian – Choose fish and chicken dishes with vegetables. Avoid big pasta dishes and garlic breads.

Chinese – Choose vegetable stir-fry, plain rice, noodles, vegetable chop suey.

French – Choose fish and poultry or vegetarian options with salad or vegetables. Avoid anything in a heavy sauce.

Mediterranean – Choose salads, vegetarian dishes, fish and chicken dishes.

Snacks

If you occasionally get hungry between meals, choose a healthy snack from the box below to boost your blood sugar and you'll resist that chocolate digestive. If you really want something sweet, choose natural foods, which contain fibre and are nutrient-rich – a flapjack, for example (which is full of fibre and nutrients such as magnesium, calcium, iron and vitamin B5) will leave you feeling sated for longer than a piece of chocolate. But if you really cannot do without the odd sweet treat, don't eat it as a snack – enjoy it at the end of your meal, as the fibre and fat from your main course will delay the sugar rush.

Good snacks

If you need to snack mid-morning and mid-afternoon, try to achieve a balance of protein and carbohydrate with each snack.
- Natural bio-yoghurt with an apple or pear
- 10 almonds with apple, pear, cherries or berries
- Oatcake biscuit with tahini, houmous or avocado guacamole
- Small handful of mixed nuts and dried fruit
- Rice cake with houmous, tahini or cottage cheese

Drinks

Remember to drink regularly — include at least eight glasses (1½ litres) of pure water a day. Herbal teas are also great for keeping you well hydrated. Avoid tea, coffee and all fizzy drinks. Health drinks, like Amé and Aqua Libra, are okay in moderation. Alcohol should be avoided for your six-week programme.

If you like your coffee, it will not be easy to stop drinking it immediately because coffee has a profound effect upon the body's biochemistry. Instead, reduce your intake gradually and drink as much water as you can to minimize the side effects. It is not unusual to get headaches and feel washed out when giving up coffee. Rest assured that it will pass — even if this seems impossible to believe after suffering for four days — and you will soon have more energy than you ever did when you relied on coffee for a pick-me-up.

MENU PLANS

	DAY 1	DAY 2	DAY 3	DAY 4	DAY 5	DAY 6	DAY 7
BREAKFAST	Yoghurt and berry smoothie *(see recipes, page 229)*	Boiled, scrambled or poached egg 1 slice rye toast with tahini spread or a thin scraping of butter Piece of fresh fruit Glass of orange juice	2 fruit kebabs *(see recipes, page 231)* Natural live bio-yoghurt	Rice cakes with cottage cheese (or marmite, houmous, or a small amount of peanut butter) Piece of fresh fruit	Bowl of natural live bio-yoghurt, tbsp of mixed seeds and diced fruit *(choose from apple, pear, banana, kiwi, peach, apricot, orange or grapefruit)* Herbal tea	Porridge oats made with rice milk (or alternative) mixed with diced dried fruit (apricots, prunes, bananas, berries, raisins) and a tbsp of flaxseeds	Porridge oats cooked with water or milk substitute, sprinkled with a tbsp of mixed seeds and raspberries Herbal tea
LUNCH	Large mixed green salad and a two-egg omelette	Mixed bean and vegetable soup *(see recipes, page 253)*, or choose from the supermarket range of ready-made fresh soups Piece of fresh fruit	Grated fresh beetroot and grated celeriac, sprinked with lemon juice and sesame seeds Natural live bio-yoghurt	Small baked potato or sweet potato *(do have a small one, as they have quite a high glycaemic index – see page 206)* Choose from fillings such as tuna, cottage cheese, baked beans, houmous and roast chicken breast Green salad	3 slices of chicken breast Green salad, made with lambs' lettuce, mange tout and sliced courgette Piece of fresh fruit	Rice cakes with cottage chesse *(try all the different varieties – such as pineapple, chives or prawn)* Natural live bio-yoghurt	Houmous with crudités *(for example, carrots, broccoli florets, baby corn, cauliflower, cucumber or celery)* Oatcakes Piece of fresh fruit
DINNER	Black-eyed bean balti *(see recipes, page 234)* Mixed salad Natural live yoghurt or fresh fruit	Chicken provençale *(see recipes, page 244)* Brown rice and salad	Pan-fried Dover sole with wilted spinach and lemon dressing *(see recipes, page 237)*	Grilled red snapper with green chillies *(see recipes, page 245)* Selection of raw vegetables	Stuffed tomatoes with chickpeas and coriander *(see recipes, page 242)* Mixed salad	Stuffed aubergines *(see recipes, page 239)*	Salmon with roasted sweet potato chips *(see recipes, page 247)* Stir-fried green vegetables of your choice

DAY 8	DAY 9	DAY 10	DAY 11	DAY 12	DAY 13	DAY 14	
Scrambled egg and smoked salmon Glass of orange juice	Breakfast smoothie *(see recipes, page 231)*	Cottage cheese on toasted rye bread *(spread with tahini or a scraping of butter if required)* Small handful of walnuts Piece of fresh fruit	Fresh fruit juice *(see recipes, page 232)* 1 boiled egg Slice of wheat-free bread Herbal tea	Wheat-free cereal such as Mesa Sunrise *(see Resources, page 260)* or millet flakes with skimmed milk and a tbsp of mixed seeds Small glass of fresh juice	Sugar-free baked beans on rye or spelt toast *(spelt is a wheat grain, but it is less allergenic than wheat)* Piece of fresh fruit	Mixed melon salad *(see recipes, page 229)* 1 tbsp of seeds	BREAKFAST
Choice of soup *(see the recipes on page 250, or choose from supermarket fresh soup ranges)* 1 slice rye bread Piece of fresh fruit	Grilled peppers Green salad Natural live bio-yoghurt	Peppered smoked mackerel, alfalfa and natural live bio-yoghurt Piece of fresh fruit	Carrot, celery and apple salad Sliced chicken breast Natural live bio-yoghurt or piece of fresh fruit	Nut and mango salad 2 tbsp cottage cheese Piece of fresh fruit	Mixed bean and vegetable soup *(see recipes, page 253)* Salad	Boiled egg 1 slice rye bread	LUNCH
Broccoli and almond risotto *(see recipes, page 235)* Chickpea, lime and coriander salad *(see recipes, page 249)*	Chicken provençale *(see recipes, page 244)* Steamed vegetables	Grilled fish of your choice Green salad Butter bean mash *(see recipes, page 248)* Piece of fresh fruit	Rich bean and vegetable stew *(see recipes, page 240)*	Oven-cooked salmon with large green salad Serving of quinoa *(cook according to packet instructions)*. Use quinoa as you would use couscous, perhaps mixing with diced, roasted vegetables or dried fruit or nuts Natural live bio-yoghurt	Pan-fried John Dory with baby bok choy *(see recipes, page 238)*	Fillet of pork with prunes *(see recipes, page 236)* Selection of vegetables	DINNER

Recipes

BREAKFAST

Breakfasts don't need to be complicated to be good for you. The simplest ingredients can deliver the nutrients you need to keep you going all morning. Try:

- Scrambled eggs made with a teaspoon of rice milk and smoked salmon. High in protein, it will help you feel alert and motivated until lunch.

- Porridge oats – the perfect complex carbohydrate. They're a great pre-training breakfast because they release energy slowly into the bloodstream. Rich in soluble fibre and pectin, oats have been shown to benefit the digestive system, hormone balance and cholesterol levels. Use a milk alternative such as soya or almond milk. You can add diced dried fruit (apricots, prunes, bananas, berries or raisins) and a tablespoon of flaxseeds. Flaxseed is rich in omega-3 oils and soluble fibre, which help carry toxins and waste products out of the body. The dried fruit provides glucose for energy, but it's also packed with nutrients. Dried apricots are a good source of iron, which is particularly important if you are putting your body through more exercise than you are used to.

- Smoothies make a fantastic start to the day. If you use yoghurt and fruit you'll get a good balance of protein and carbohydrate to help balance your blood sugar. Think about adding some ground seeds, too – packed with essential fats and zinc, they're a great energy-booster and can help balance hormones and improve your skin.

Natural yoghurt and berry smoothie

1 mug mixed berries (you can use frozen berries if fresh ones are not in season)
1 banana
4 tbsp natural live bio-yoghurt
Large tumbler of ice
Rice or soya milk (optional)

1. Put the fruit and ice in the liquidizer and give it a quick burst. Add the natural yoghurt and liquidize. Add rice or soya milk to adjust the consistency.

Alternatives:
Experiment with combinations of peach and strawberry, pineapple and mango.

Mixed melon salad

Packed with vitamin C, this breakfast is a good immune booster. All forms of melon are also stimulating for the kidneys, so it's a good detoxifier.

1 large slice red watermelon
¼ orange cantaloupe melon
¼ yellow melon
Sprigs of mint
A few seedless green grapes

1. Dice the melon or scoop into balls using a melon baller. Place in a bowl with the grapes, and garnish with the mint.

For a breakfast on the run

Of course we don't all have the luxury of time to prepare and eat a leisurely breakfast everyday. However, it is still important that you have something more substantial than a croissant at the station. Why not try:

- Trophy seed or fruit bars (available in Waitrose, Sainsbury's and other supermarkets and health food stores)
- Ready-made smoothies (available from most station shops or cafés)
- Pot of natural bio-yoghurt and a piece of fruit
- Fresh fruit with a few nuts
- Snack-sized bag of seeds (see Resources, page 260) and a banana

Alternatives to milk and cream:
- Natural live bio-yoghurt
- Oat milk
- Rice milk
- Soya milk

Fruit kebabs

SERVES 4

This is a light, cleansing breakfast, packed with antioxidant nutrients to give your immune system a boost. The yoghurt adds some protein to make this breakfast more sustaining. Be sure to choose live bio-yoghurt because of the health-promoting benefits of the beneficial bacteria.

3 apricots
2 kiwi fruits
1 nectarine
1 peach
1 banana
8 strawberries
1 tbsp honey
1 tsp grated lemon rind
2 tsp lemon juice
Pinch of cinnamon
7 oz (200 g) natural live bio-yoghurt

1. Chop the fruit into chunky pieces and thread onto small wooden skewers. Mix together the lemon juice, honey and cinnamon and brush over the kebabs. Put the kebabs under a hot grill for 2 minutes, turning regularly. Serve hot, with natural yoghurt.

Juice Cocktails

Fresh juices are a delicious, refreshing way to get lots of nutrients without lots of calories. Here are some great juice cocktails to try:

- The immune booster: ginger, beetroot and carrot. You could also add grapefruit-seed extract or propolis to your juice of choice
- For the heart and circulation: orange, red pepper, alfalfa and coriander
- To help PMS symptoms: fennel, pineapple, spinach and ginger
- The energy-booster: cucumber, celery and beetroot, or apple, carrot and ginger – they are high in nutrients and low in calories
- The detox: apple, spinach and onion juice (you can also add a clove of garlic and a teaspoon of psyllium husks), or add a few drops to milk thistle tincture to your juice of choice
- To help with constipation: add a teaspoon of psyllium husk powder to your juice of choice

MAIN MEALS

Black-eyed bean Balti

SERVES 4

11 oz (300 g) black-eyed beans
4 bay leaves
3 cardamom pods
3 garlic cloves, crushed
½ tsp ground turmeric
1½ oz (40 g) fresh root ginger, grated
2 dried red chillies, crushed and de-seeded
3 tbsp olive oil
1 tsp ground cumin
3½ oz (100 g) low-fat natural yoghurt
3 onions, finely chopped
4 tomatoes
3 sprigs of coriander, chopped, to garnish

1. Soak the beans for 12 hours in cold water, then cook them slowly for 1 hour in boiling water, with the bay leaves, cardamom, turmeric and half the crushed garlic, until tender. When cooked, drain and reserve the liquid.
2. In a large, heavy-based saucepan, cook the onions, tomatoes, ginger, chillies and remaining garlic in olive oil for 5 minutes. Add the ground cumin, black-eyed beans, yoghurt and some of the reserved liquid. Cook for another 5 minutes until the sauce thickens. Garnish with fresh, chopped coriander and serve with rice.

Recipe by Susan Clark

Broccoli and almond risotto

SERVES 6

7 oz (200 g) broccoli
1 red onion, finely diced
1 garlic clove, chopped
6 tbsp olive oil
11 oz (300 g) Arborio rice
1¾ pt (1 l) vegetable stock
6 fresh sage leaves, chopped
Freshly ground black pepper
4 tbsp almond cream
3½ oz (100 g) blanched almonds
2 oz (50 g) Parmesan cheese (optional)

1. Blanch (cook briefly) the broccoli in a pan of boiling water.
2. In another large pan, cook the diced onion and chopped garlic in the olive oil until tender. Add the rice and stir for 2 minutes to coat all the grains. Cover the rice with a little of the hot vegetable stock and cook gently for 10 minutes, stirring frequently.
3. Add the broccoli, sage and seasoning. Gradually add more stock as the rice absorbs all the liquid. Continue to cook until the rice is tender (it should take about 25 minutes in total).
4. When the rice is cooked, add the almond cream, whole almonds and Parmesan cheese (if using). Stir and check seasoning.

Alternatives: as a variation use other nuts or different blanched vegetables, for example, asparagus or green beans.

Recipe by Susan Clark

Fillet of pork with prunes

SERVES 6

18 prunes
36 oz (1 kg) pork fillet
3 oz (90 g) walnuts
3 oz (90 g) almonds
3 oz (90 g) hazelnuts
3½ oz (100 g) honey
4 tbsp cider vinegar
½ pt (300 ml) chicken stock
Freshly ground black pepper
2 oz (50 g) white flour (for coating the pork)
3 tbsp olive oil
1 bunch of fresh chives, chopped, to garnish

1. Soak the prunes in water for 8 hours. Trim the pork fillets and cut widthways into 2.5 cm discs. Gently crush the nuts. Drain the prunes and cut them in half.
2. In a saucepan, heat the honey until it turns to a caramel colour. Add the vinegar with the chicken stock. Season and reduce the sauce until it becomes syrupy and coats the back of the spoon. Complete the sauce by adding the nuts and the prunes. Put to one side.
3. Coat each piece of pork in flour and cook in hot olive oil until golden brown on both sides. Allow 4 minutes cooking time on each side. Season and serve. Present the pork covered with the prune sauce garnished with chopped chives. Serve with a selection of vegetables.

Recipe by Susan Clark

Bodydoctor

Pan-fried Dover sole fillets with wilted spinach and lemon dressing

SERVES 4

4 Dover sole fillets
12 tbsp olive oil
14 oz (400 g) baby spinach
7 oz (200 g) green beans (topped and tailed)
3 tbsp lemon juice
2 tbsp water
Salt

1. Bring a pan of water to the boil and season with salt. Add the prepared green beans and cook until tender.
2. Make the lemon dressing by mixing 9 tbsp olive oil, the lemon juice, water and salt together until emulsified.
3. Pour 3 tbsp olive oil into a non-stick pan and heat on a stove. When hot, add the Dover sole fillets. Allow to colour on one side, turn them over once this is done and season with salt and pepper.
4. To serve, wilt the spinach in a little water and salt. Once cooked, drain and put in the middle of a plate. Drain the beans and scatter around the spinach. Place the fish on top and drizzle on the lemon dressing.

Recipe by Jean-Christophe Novelli

Pan-fried fillet of John Dory, spiced carrot juice and baby bok choy

SERVES 4

4 John Dory fillets (skinned)

4 bunches of baby Dutch carrots

1 tsp cumin powder

½ bay leaf

15 tbsp olive oil

7 oz (200 g) baby spinach

1 baby bok choy cut in half

4 new potatoes

¾ pt (400 ml) water

1 squeeze of lemon

Salt and pepper

1. Peel, top and tail the baby carrots and then pass them through a juicer so as to extract the juice only. Keep to one side.
2. Wash the baby spinach and cut the baby bok choy in half lengthways. Wash the new potatoes and place in a suitable size pan and then cover with water and add salt. Bring to boil and simmer for 10–15 minutes, depending on size. Allow to cool in the liquid. Once cold, peel and slice into 1 cm-wide slices.
3. Warm a small pan on the stove. Add the cumin and singe for 1 minute, then allow to cool slightly. Add the carrot juice and bay leaf and simmer for 4 minutes. Take off the heat and whisk in 2 tbsp of olive oil.
4. Take the bok choy and cook in simmering salted water for approximately 6–7 minutes.
5. Place a non-stick pan on the stove and add a little olive oil. When hot, add the fish to it followed by the sliced new potatoes. Wilt the baby spinach with olive oil and season with salt and pepper. By this time the fish should be a nice golden brown colour. Turn along with the potatoes, season and take the potatoes out. Add a little lemon juice. Warm the carrot juice. Drain all the vegetables and arrange on a plate. Place the fish on top and drizzle the sauce around.

Recipe by Jean-Christophe Novelli

Stuffed aubergines

SERVES 6

7 oz (200 g) raisins
6 aubergines
Juice of 2 lemons
7 tbsp olive oil
5 large onions, finely chopped
5 tbsp chopped fresh flat-leafed parsley
10 tomatoes, skinned, de-seeded and chopped
5 garlic cloves, crushed
1 pinch of cayenne pepper
1 sprig of fresh thyme
3 bay leaves
Freshly ground black pepper

1. Soak the raisins in a bowl of warm water. Halve the aubergines lengthways and then extract and dice the flesh without piercing the skins. Mix the flesh with the juice of 1 lemon.
2. Heat the olive oil and sauté the diced aubergines, onions, parsley, tomatoes, crushed garlic, cayenne pepper, thyme and bay leaves. Season and cook for 30 minutes. Drain the raisins and add to the mixture when it is cooked.
3. Place the empty aubergine skins in an oven-proof dish. Stuff them with the vegetable mixture and cook in a pre-heated oven (160°C/325°F/Gas 3) for 1½ hours. Squeeze over the juice of the second lemon before serving.

Alternatives: to make this a meat dish, add 10½ oz (300g) of lean minced lamb to the stuffing with the raisins.

Recipe by Susan Clark

Rich bean and vegetable stew

SERVES 4

Pulses are one of the great superfoods – high in protein and complex carbohydrate, rich in minerals and fibre, a good source of B complex vitamins and very low in fat. Pulses make a great choice for a pre or post-exercise meal. The herbs and garlic can help counter the flatulence often associated with eating pulses.

4 oz (100 g) dried porcini mushrooms
3 tbsp olive oil
8 oz (225 g) large open mushrooms
2 carrots, finely diced
1 sweet potato, diced
8 oz (225 g) fine green beans, chopped
½ tbsp dried thyme
½ tbsp dried sage
2 cloves crushed garlic
1½ pints (900 ml) vegetable stock
Salt and black pepper
8 oz (225g) broad beans (you can use frozen beans)
10 oz (300 g) can cannellini beans
8 oz (225 g) can flageolet beans

1. Cover the porcini with 1 pint (600 ml) of boiling water and leave to soak for 20 minutes.
2. Heat the oil in a large saucepan, then add the fresh mushrooms, carrots, potatoes and green beans. Stir-fry gently for 3–4 minutes until slightly softened.
3. Add the thyme, sage, garlic, porcini mushrooms in their soaking liquid, stock and seasoning. Bring to the boil and simmer uncovered for 20 minutes until the vegetables are tender.
4. Stir in the broad beans and simmer for a further 10 minutes or until tender. Drain and rinse the cannellini and flageolet beans. Add to the mixture and simmer for 2–3 minutes to heat through.

Recipe by Colin Spencer

Ways with stir-fry

Stir-frying is an excellent, quick way to cook your vegetables because it minimizes nutrient loss. You can stir-fry all vegetables, but be inventive – try bok choi, broccoli, carrots, mange tout, peppers, bean sprouts, onion, and garlic. Cook the vegetables in a splash of olive oil. To keep up the nutrient level, add a tablespoon of water to the oil and steam-cook the vegetables by covering the pan or wok with a lid. Try the following flavourings to spice up the taste:

- 1 tbsp soy sauce
- Juice of 1 lemon
- Splash of sesame oil
- Clove of crushed garlic

Stuffed tomatoes with chickpeas and coriander

SERVES 2

This is a great light meal to give your immune system a boost and also provides enough complex carbohydrate to set you up for your exercise routine.

2 slices rye bread
4 large tomatoes
1 clove garlic
4 oz (100 g) tinned chickpeas, rinsed and drained
Juice of 1 lemon
1 tbsp olive oil
1 red onion, finely chopped
¼ tsp cayenne pepper
1 tsp ground cumin
1 tsp ground coriander
4 tsp fresh coriander, chopped
Salt and pepper to taste

1. Pre-heat the oven to 160°C/325°F, and bake the bread in the oven for 20 minutes until crisp. Process in a food processor to make breadcrumbs.
2. Increase the oven temperature to 200°C/400°F. Slice off the tops of the tomatoes and scoop out the flesh and seeds. Place the shells upside down on some kitchen roll to drain.
3. Put the insides and tops into a food processor with the garlic, chickpeas and lemon juice. Blend to a purée.
4. Heat the oil and cook the onion with the cayenne pepper, cumin and coriander for 4–5 minutes until softened. Mix with the tomato, breadcrumbs, fresh coriander and seasoning.
5. Spoon the mixture into the tomato shells and cook for 20 minutes until tender.

Recipe by Colin Spencer (Tesco Recipe Collection)

Ratatouille

SERVES 2

A classic dish to keep up your vegetable intake, providing complex carbohydrate for energy, fibre for the digestive system and packed with immune-boosting nutrients.

Choose a selection of these vegetables:
aubergine, courgettes, red, yellow or green peppers, fennel
5 tomatoes
2 onions, chopped
2 cloves garlic, sliced
Juice of half a lemon
Chilli flakes
Black pepper
Dried oregano

1. Cook the garlic with onions, chilli flakes and vegetables (excluding tomatoes) for 5 minutes. Add the tomatoes, lemon juice and seasoning and simmer for a further 10–15 minutes until all the vegetables are soft.

Recipe by Susan Clark

Chicken Provençale

SERVES 2

This comforting meal is ideal after exercise. Chicken is a low-fat source of protein and it's also packed with zinc for energy, healthy skin and optimum immune function. Buy organic if you can, as it is free from hormones commonly used in chicken farming.

3¼ lb (1.5 kg) chicken legs and thighs, skinned
6 tbsp olive oil
2 large chopped onions
5 cloves garlic, chopped
3 large shallots, chopped
18 oz (500 g) red peppers, cut into strips
18 oz (500 g) tomatoes, chopped
4 fl oz (100 ml) white wine
1 sprig oregano
1 sprig thyme
2 bay leaves, crushed
1 pinch cayenne pepper
Freshly ground black pepper
5¼ oz (155 g) pitted green olives
4 oz (100 g) pitted black olives
5 fresh basil leaves, chopped

1. Brown the chicken pieces in olive oil for 5 minutes. Remove from the pan and set aside.
2. In the same saucepan gently cook the onions, garlic and shallots until tender. Add the pepper strips, chopped tomatoes, wine, oregano, thyme, bay leaves and cayenne pepper.
3. Return the chicken pieces to the pan. Season, cover and cook very slowly, over a low heat for 1 hour. Add the olives, and cook for a further 20 minutes, before sprinkling with chopped fresh basil.
4. Serve with brown rice and steamed vegetables.

Recipe by Susan Clark

Grilled red snapper with green chillies and coconut

SERVES 6 *(as a light meal)*

Most of us don't eat nearly enough fish. Oily fish, like the mackerel or sardines that can be used in this recipe, are a very rich source of omega-3 essential fatty acids, which are vital for a healthy heart, immune and endocrine system.

6 red snappers, 6 mackerel or 6 sardines

For the paste
1 large onion, roughly chopped
5 garlic cloves
5 fresh green chillies
3 oz (75 g) fresh coconut flesh
4 tbsp fresh coriander
1 tsp ground cumin
Juice of 2 limes
1 in (2.5 cm) fresh root ginger
1 teaspoon salt

1. Slash the fish 3 or 4 times diagonally on each side.
2. Put all the paste ingredients in a food processor and blend.
3. Baste the fish with the paste and grill for 5–7 minutes on each side, under a medium heat, until the green sauce begins to bubble and the fish flesh flakes.
4. Serve with a selection of raw vegetables.

Recipe by Susan Clark

ACCOMPANIMENTS

Sweet potato chips

SERVES 4

Sweet potatoes are better for your blood sugar balance than normal potatoes, and they are also rich in the anti-cancer, anti-oxidant, beta carotene.

22 oz (650 g) sweet potatoes
2 cloves garlic
1 tbsp chopped rosemary
3 tbsp olive oil

1. Cut the sweet potatoes into chips.
2. Mix chopped garlic, chopped rosemary and olive oil. Spread the oil and garlic mixture over the potato.
3. Cook in an oven pre-heated to 230°C/450°F for 25 minutes, or until soft.

Recipe by Susan Clark

Butter bean mash

SERVES 4

Like other pulses, butter beans are a rich source of protein, minerals and fibre. Use this mash to accompany meat or fish and a big green salad for a post-exercise meal.

14 oz (400 g) dried butter beans
10 fresh sage leaves
1 sprig fresh rosemary
½ medium carrot
½ medium onion
4 tbsp olive oil
5 tsp balsamic vinegar
Black pepper

1. Soak the butter beans overnight.
2. Cook in a pan of water with the sage, rosemary, carrot and onion for 1–1½ hours until tender. Discard the herbs, carrot and onions, and mash three-quarters of the beans with some of the cooking juice. Add the balsamic vinegar and olive oil, and season to taste. Add the remainder of the beans, leaving them unmashed to provide texture.

Recipe by Susan Clark

Salads

Try to have a least one salad every day. Sprinkle your salads with nuts or seeds and go for delicious dressings made from olive oil, sesame oil or an essential oil mix such as Udo's Choice (see Resources, page 260); add garlic, balsamic vinegar, and lime or lemon juice for a refreshing taste. Fresh herbs such as basil, parsley, mint and coriander add interesting flavours and are packed with nutrients and immune-boosting compounds.

Try:

- Rocket, pear and walnut
- Fig, lambs lettuce and a small slice of Parma ham (with excess fat removed)
- Lettuce, mange tout (raw) and cold cooked petit pois
- Red and white kidney beans, tomatoes, red and green peppers (dressed with olive oil and balsamic vinegar) with guacamole. For the guacamole, peel and finely chop half a clove of garlic, add the flesh of an avocado and mash together. Add salt, fresh lime juice and Tabasco sauce to taste
- Chickpea, onion, red pepper and garlic with fresh lime juice and coriander
- Roasted peppers chopped on bed of rocket. Garnish with fresh basil and sage
- Bean sprouts, Chinese leaves, cold shiitake mushrooms, sugar snap peas, seeded chillies and finely chopped red pepper. Dress with sesame oil, lime juice and crushed garlic.

SOUPS

Sweet spicy tomato gaspacho

SERVES 4

40 oz (1.1 kg) vine ripe plum tomatoes
1 oz (25 g) Spanish onions
1¾ oz (50 g) cucumber
2 cloves garlic
7½ oz (215 g) red peppers
Salt and cayenne pepper
1 tsp white wine vinegar
Thyme (to season)

For the basil, avocado and mint ice cubes:
¼ pt (150 ml) vegetable stock
8 fresh basil leaves
2 sprigs of mint
¾ avocado
2 drops lemon juice
2 drops Tabasco sauce
1 drop Worcester Sauce

1. Cut the tomatoes in half lengthways and season with garlic, thyme, salt and white pepper. Place the tomatoes on a tray and dry in a low oven at 80°C until they are moist (not thoroughly dried out).
2. Once dried, remove the thyme and garlic. Peel the onions and garlic and deseed the peppers. Chop to about 2 cm and dice along with the tomatoes, then place in a bowl with the cucumber, cayenne pepper and white wine vinegar and marinade for 12 hours. Blitz and pass. Season as required before placing in the fridge to cool completely before serving.
3. Meanwhile, prepare the basil, avocado and mint ice cubes. Bring the vegetable stock to simmer and infuse with basil and mint. Allow to cool. Peel and dice the avocado and roll the diced avocado around in the lemon juice. Once the stock liquid is cooled, pass through a fine sieve. Blitz the avocado and add the stock to it, adding Tabasco and Worcester sauce. Freeze the liquid in little ice-cube containers
4. Serve the gaspacho in a cold glass with the basil, avocado and mint ice cubes.

Recipe by Jean-Christophe Novelli

Shiitake soup

SERVES 6

This is the perfect soup if you are recovering from a cold or flu. Shiitake mushrooms contain an immune-boosting chemical called lentinan, and have been used for centuries in traditional Chinese medicine.

9 oz (250 g) smoked tofu, diced
4½ oz (125 g) shiitake mushrooms, sliced
4 tbsp fresh coriander
Bunch of watercress
1 medium red chilli, sliced, to garnish

For the stock:
2 dried chillies, chopped
1½ oz (35 g) tamarind pulp
Kaffir lime leaves
1 onion, chopped
1 stalk lemon grass
1 in (2.5 cm) fresh root ginger, grated
1¾ pint (1 litre) water

1. Boil all the stock ingredients together for 10 minutes. Drain through a fine sieve, reserving the liquid and discarding the contents of the sieve.
2. Stir-fry the tofu in a wok for a few minutes, then add the stock, mushrooms and coriander. Boil for 5 minutes.
3. Add the watercress and cook for another 2 minutes.
4. Garnish with the sliced chilli, and serve hot.

Recipe by Susan Clark

Mixed bean and vegetable soup

SERVES 4

This soup is a hearty combination of vegetables and pulses, full of antioxidants and fibre, and good to eat pre- or post-exercise.

2 tbsp olive oil
1 onion, finely chopped
2 cloves garlic
1 sweet potato
1 carrot
2 tsp cumin seeds
1½ pints (900 ml) vegetable stock
2 sticks celery
1 large courgette
5 oz (150 g) fine green beans, chopped
15 oz (420 g) can butter beans
14 oz (400 g) can tomatoes
Black pepper

1. Heat the oil and add the onion, garlic, potato, carrot and cumin. Cook for 5 minutes, stirring occasionally, until the vegetables have softened.
2. Add the stock, celery and courgette and bring to the boil. Cover and simmer for 10 minutes or until the celery and courgette are tender.
3. Stir in the green beans, butter beans and chopped tomatoes. Season. Simmer uncovered for 5 minutes before serving.

Recipe by Emma Patmore (Tesco Recipe Collection)

A Last Word

By this stage you are hopefully encouraged to take control of your health and well-being. I have always been aware that my clients have initially been attracted to Bodydoctor Fitness because of the aesthetic transformations that we are recognized for. However, losing between 1 and 3 sizes and ridding yourself of unwanted and unnecessary body fat are just peripheral points. The true depth of our work is in helping to restore your body to a state close to optimum health. You have now been armed with the information and knowledge, but this is useless without application.

Our aim is to bring fitness into your home and everyday life. If you don't have the tools i.e., weights, stability balls, ab-rollers and benches, we will help you acquire them at hugely advantageous prices delivered to your door. Reebok Fitness and a number of other suppliers have agreed to supply readers with all the products necessary to turn this book into action at our website www.bodydoctor.com.

You can see some of these exercises come to life in 2-minute videos on our website. Sit in front of your screen, watch it and then get on the floor and do it. It really is that simple. There is a video and DVD of both the home and gym programmes available to order from the website, as well as weekly nutritional and holistic health newsletters. You can also carry out over 53 interactive fitness and health assessments.

To book a one-on-one fitness training course of 20 sessions call:
London – 020 7586 6222; Bournemouth – 01202 318142
Mauritius – Le Prince Maurice hotel, 00 230 413 9100, www.princemaurice.com

Additional members of the bodydoctor holistic team are:
Phillip Beach: Osteopathy, Naturopathy and Acupuncture
Philip Hochhauser: Traditional Chinese Medicine and Acupuncture
Sean Durkan: Osteopathy
Kevin Bell: Osteopathy and Pilates
Amanda Moore, Gudrun Jonsson and Vicki Edgson: Nutritional Therapy
Brian Caplan: Homeopathy
David Holland: Podiatry

Details of this team and booking facilities can be found on the website.

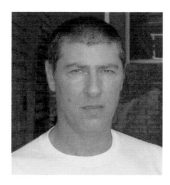

The training techniques I use are in complete contrast to the same old sequences that have been churned out time and again over the past 60 years. You have probably tried many other methods to no avail. My programme is very simple and I've always found that simplicity usually equates to beauty and efficiency. Just follow it to the letter and see the results for yourself. Everything you need to know has been included, anything that is useless to you has been left out.

You can't get fit, slim and healthy by just reading about it. All you need to do is DO IT.

If you suffer from weight-related problems you probably think that you have a mountain to climb. The reality is that you only have a slope to negotiate. Anything is difficult if you do not know how to do it properly. You now have the information. Your results can be as good as you want them to be. Do it with a good heart. Look forward and enjoy.

Send us detailed feedback — what you've achieved and how you've got on — by email to feedback@bodydoctor.com. The best email each month will win a complementary one-to-one training session at the Bodydoctor premises closest to you.

GOOD LUCK!

RECOMMENDED READING, BIBLIOGRAPHY AND RESOURCES

Bodydoctor®

Recommended Reading

The X-Factor Diet, Leslie Kenton, Random House 2002

Nutrition Practitioner, The ONC Journal, volume 4 issue 1, August 2002

Life without Bread. How a low-carbohydrate diet can save your life, Allan, Christian, B, Lutz, Wolfgang. Keats Publishing, Los Angeles, 2000

Optimum Sports Nutrition, Michael Colgan, Advanced Research Press, 1993

The New Nutrition, Michael Colgan, Apple Tree Publishing, 1996

Fats that Heal, Fats that Kill, Udo Erasmus, Alive Books, 1998

Bibliography

1 Report of cancer incidence and prevalence projections, East Anglican Cancer Intelligence Unit, University of Cambridge. Macmillan Cancer Relief, June 1977

2 Hodges s et al. *Biofactors* 9:365–370, 1999

3 *New England Journal of Medicine,* March 14 2002. 346:802–810 854–855

4 *Fats That Heal, Fats that Kill* Dr Udo Erasmus, Alive Books, 1993

5 Eaton, SB and Konner, MJ. Palaeolithic nutrition. *New England Journal of Medicine,* 1985. 312: 283–289.

6 Eaton, SB and Konner, MJ. Palaeolithic nutrition. *New England Journal of Medicine,* 1985. 312: 283–289.

7 J. Yudkin et al. Effects of high dietary sugar. *British Journal of Medicine* 281, November 22, 1980, pp 1396.

8 A Koziovsky et al. Effects of diets high in simple sugars on urinary chromium losses. *Metabolism* 35, June 1986 pp 515–518

9 J Goldman et al. Behavioural effects of sucrose on pre-school children. *Journal of Abnormal Child Psychology* 14 1986, 565–577

10 A Sanchez et al. Role of sugars in human neutrophilic phagocytosis. *American Journal of Clinical Nutrition,* November 1973 pp 1180-1184

11 UK National Food Survey 1995

12 MAFF (1994). The dietary and nutritional survey of British adults – further analysis. HMSO, London, UK

13 Schectman G et al. Ascorbic acid requirements for smokers: Analysis of a population survey. *American Journal of Clinical Nutrition* 1991 vol 53: pp 1466–1470

14 *Journal of the American Medical Association*

15 Daily InScight. A Better Whey to Heal? Academic Press, 1997

16 Bounous G et al. The immunoenhancing properties of dietary whey protein concentrate. *Clinical and Investigative Medicine* 11:271-278, 1988

17 Michael N Sawka, PhD et al. Abstract from NIH workshop: The role of dietary supplements for physically active people

18 Sawka et al. Physiological consequences of hypohydration: body water redistribution, exercise performance and temp. regulation. *Medicine and Science in Sports and Exercise* 1992; 24: 657–70

19 Medical Research Council: Report for MPs, July 10 2000

20 BNF published report: Metabolic syndrome new research underway, 2003

21 Serdula et al. Prevalence of attempting weight loss and strategies for controlling weight. JAMA, 1999; 282:113538

22 *Optimum Sports Nutrition,* Dr Michael Colgan. Advanced Research Press, 1993

23 A randomised trial of a low-carbohydrate diet for obesity. *New England Journal of Medicine,* 2003; 348:2082–90

24 A low-carbohydrate as compared with a low-fat diet in severe obesity. *New England Journal of Medicine* 2003; 348:2074–81

25 G Evans et al. The effects of chromium picolinate on insulin controlled parameters in humans, *International Journal of Biosocial and Medical Research* 1989. Vol 1. No 2: 163–180

26 Gorostiaga et al. Decrease in respiratory quotient during exercise following L-carnitine supplementation. *International Jurnal of Sports Medicine* 1989;10:169–174

27 D Clouatre and M Rousenbaaum. The diet and health benefits of HCA. Keats Publishing, 1994

Source of recipes

The Sunday Times Vitality Cookbook, Susan Clark, HarperCollins *Publishers* 1999, the UK's leading journalist, author and broadcaster specializing in natural health.
Visit her website, www.whatreallyworks.co.uk. Recipes devised with Erick Muzard.
Shiitake soup
Red snapper and green chillies (variation on Grilled mackerel with green sauce)
Butter bean mash (part of a recipe)
Chicken provençale

Mainly Vegetables, Colin Spencer, Brilliant Books Ltd. Published for Tesco.
Stuffed tomatoes with chickpeas and coriander
Variation on Rich bean and vegetable stew

Fast Family Meals, Emma Patmore, Brilliant Books. Published for Tesco.
Mixed vegetable and bean soup

Resources

Supplements

Biocare Ltd
Lakeside
180 Lifford Lane
Kings Norton
Birmingham
B30 3NU
Tel: 0102 433 3727
E-mail: biocare@biocare.co.uk

Nutri Ltd
Meridian House
Botany Business Park
Whaley Bridge
High Peak
SK23 7DQ
Tel: 0800 212742
E-mail: orders@nutri.co.uk

Solgar Vitamins Ltd
Aldbury
Tring
Herts
HP23 5PT
Tel: 01442 890355

The Nutri Centre
7 Park Crescent
London
W1N 3HF
Tel: 020 7436 5122

Gluten-free Foods

Nutritional Advice
British Association of Nutritional therapists
21 Old Gloucester Street
London
WC1N 3XX
Tel: 0870 6061284
Website: www.bant.co.uk

Institute for Optimum Nutrition
Blades Court
Deodar Road
London
SW15 2NU
Tel: 0181 877 9993
Website: www.optimumnutrition.co.uk

INDEX

Bodydoctor®